Whole: A Leg Up On Life

Kendra Herber

Author's Note:

In order to write this book, I relied upon candid, familial conversations especially regarding my younger years in order to reproduce events in which I have no memory. Later information is all depicted as I recall it and is as factual as memories can be many years after the fact. To maintain their anonymity, some names have been changed to protect their privacy.

Preface

When you hear the word amputee, what comes to mind? No matter what the image is, it's safe to say that almost everyone pictures a body part that is *missing*. But, what if our perception could change? What if, when people envision an amputee, they instead see beauty, strength, and courage? This concept is what inspired me to write this book. It is my hope that, through reading this, people begin to see what amputees have gained rather than focusing on what they've lost. The more we learn about each other, the more sensitivity we gain.

I know that every amputee's story is different, so at no point do I want readers to make assumptions or generalizations that all amputees feel a certain way or react the same way that I did. But, maybe by hearing my story, people can gain insight on *one* amputee's perspective and better relate to others that they might encounter throughout their lives. My story isn't like some of the more well-known amputee stories that make their way to the media. It didn't involve illness, an accident, or trauma. In fact, that's probably what has held me back from writing this book for all these years. In comparison to other amputees' shocking stories of survival, would mine seem trivial?

However, I've come to realize that my story matters, and it shouldn't be overlooked. Congenital amputees like me, who have a limb that doesn't form correctly or is missing at birth, have had a *lifetime* of ups and downs. Much of our daily grind goes unnoticed and isn't often discussed because people assume we've "got it figured out" since it happened so long ago. However, that's certainly not the case. I've spent over three decades trying to adjust to being an amputee. Just when I figure out one problem, another presents itself.

It took me a long time to identify as an amputee and fully embrace the culture. Being an amputee is part of who I am, but it is not *only* who I am. Just as I am a mother, wife, and teacher, I am an amputee. I have learned to love my "different appearance" and what some may deem to be my physical "flaw" or "limitation." I hope that you too can love yourself, find your inner strength, and see the humor in the bad times like I have learned to do. For it's only once those things are achieved that one truly becomes *whole*.

Whole:

They call me:
    Disadvantaged, dismissed, disabled
    Hindered, hampered, handicapped
    Impeded, impaired, invalid
    Limited, languished, lame
But, their labels don't define me. I choose my identity:
    Blessed, boundless, beautiful
    Satisfied, self-sufficient, strong
    Courageous, confident, complete
Their eyes see me as broken,
but I've never been more whole

-Kendra Herber

Chapter 1

The Prognosis

Like every expectant mother, my mom, Gail Garman, laid on the hospital bed hoping for the birthing process to be over and anticipating that joyous moment when her perfect baby would enter the world. But, her fairy tale didn't go quite as planned. You see, I was not perfect—I was deformed, in the most basic sense of the word. Because ultrasounds in 1985 weren't nearly as detailed and precise as they are today, my birth defect was a complete surprise to everyone. Talk about being blind sighted! If only they would have had time to mentally prepare, to come up with a plan...

Instead, my parents unsuspectingly awaited the nurses and doctor to shout out the same phrase they did when my older sister was born: "10 fingers and 10 toes," but all they heard was silence. They didn't think much of it at the time. Why wouldn't I be ok? Their naivety didn't allow them to do anything other than think optimistically. That is, of course, until my dad, Tim, looked down and saw what he thought to be my pinky toe on my right foot curled under a bit. The nurse's words interrupted his puzzled thoughts: "We have a problem, but it's minor. Her right foot doesn't seem to have developed all the way. We'll have the orthopedic doctor come talk to you in a bit, but it seems minor," she repeated, hoping, in vain, to settle their nerves.

My parents didn't know which emotions to feel: elation or disappointment. *Minor problem? Just how minor? How could this have happened?* Questions swirled their minds, too jumbled to be articulated.

Knowing that the nurses knew more than they did, they decided to momentarily suppress their anxiety and questions. Instead, they soaked up every second of the post-birth events. My parents reveled in the new baby smell, how big I was (at 8 pounds, 10 ounces), how much jet-black hair I had, and the delightful baby coos that I made. For those moments, I could have been any other baby in the world; I was *normal*. However, those were fleeting feelings that were soon squandered.

The next day, the orthopedic surgeon came into their hospital room to discuss "the issue" in more depth. My parents were already exhausted from the eight-hour labor the day before and lack of sleep due to newborn feeding demands, but they tried their best to focus intently on what the doctor told them. He shared that he wanted to run some tests in order to get more information.

Before long, I was being rolled away to their lab to have x-rays taken. It confirmed what the doctor suspected—I didn't have an ankle joint. Upon further examination, they told my parents that all of the following things were wrong on my right side: I was missing my fibula bone, my foot was missing several bones and was turned outward, and I only had my three biggest toes. On my left side, my hip was dislocated. They wanted my parents to be realistic about my prognosis. "I don't want to give you false hope, Mr. and Mrs. Garman," the doctor began. "If I'm being honest, Kendra might have a hard time walking and will likely never be able to run."

My parents didn't have much time to process the deflating news because the next thing they knew, the medical staff sprang into action. Their hands deftly began wrapping bandages around both of my legs to create two matching casts. Because of my left hip dislocation, I needed a cast on that leg too. The one on my right leg was put on in hopes of strengthening the tendons to keep my foot in place so it wouldn't just flop around. The doctors placed a horizontal, metal bar between my two casts at the knee joint so that I couldn't move my hip and dislocate it further. My parents were told that the casts needed to stay on for four to six weeks.

In the privacy of the hospital room, my parents were finally able to utter their true concerns, free from judgement: "Our daughter won't be like the other kids. She's handicapped. She won't ever get married. She'll have to live with us forever. How are we going to afford the medical expenses?" My dad spit out all these fears in rapid succession, unrestrained. His thoughts jumped to the extremes and only focused on the worst-case scenario while my mom somehow stayed calm and collected.

Not long after, the nurse came into my hospital room to deliver a floral arrangement from my dad's work. A gift that should have provided joy did just the opposite. It wasn't so much the flowers themselves that elicited the negative response but the vase that they were housed in. Ironically, the vase was shaped in the normal cylindrical fashion, but the bottom had two baby feet on it. Upon seeing the feet, my parents both lost it. It upset them terribly having such an evident reminder of what I was missing.

In hopes of getting her mind off it, my mom laid back on the rollaway bed that the hospital had provided her to sleep on. She closed her eyes and took a short nap. Moments after waking, her eyes came back to the dreaded vase. But, this time, it looked a bit different. There was now masking tape over the last two toes on the right foot. My mom was confused for a second, but when she looked over at my dad, he was smiling smugly at her.

Suddenly, she knew. "You did this, didn't you?" asked my mom. She could barely get the question out she was laughing so hard.

"Maybe..." my dad said. He was always worried about making other people happy, so it brought him joy to make my mom laugh. However, he often forgot about his own well-being, suppressing his emotions until they had no other choice but to escape. No matter how much humor he tried to add to mask the sadness or how tough he tried to act, sooner or later, the floodgates opened.

Unable to control his emotions, my dad fled not only the room, but the hospital itself. He raced straight to his parents' small, three-bedroom house that twelve members of his family used to occupy and told them the foreboding news through unrestrained tears. But, instead of the sympathy that he was expecting and maybe even needing, my grandpa uttered the phrase, "If you treat her like an invalid, she'll become one" in his frank, matter-of-fact demeanor. My grandpa Walt had eight other kids, so he didn't have time to devote to niceties. My dad respected my grandpa and looked up to him like any other boy does his father.

When Grandpa Walt spoke, people listened. So, when he ordered my dad to get back to the hospital and treat me exactly like he did my older sister, he did exactly that. The advice was easier to swallow despite its frankness because deep down, my dad knew that Grandpa Walt was right.

Unfortunately, that was one of the last pieces of advice my dad ever got from him. My grandpa died shortly thereafter due to complications from shingles. Because of my age, I don't even remember him. I only remember what he looked like from seeing the pictures in our family photo albums. I wish I could recall the man's face who changed the course of my life. Because my dad rarely went to him for advice, it made Grandpa Walt's words stand out as being even more pivotal. At the time, my grandpa couldn't have known that his wise words would have the lasting impact on me that they did. But even if he didn't, I am still reaping their benefit to this day. Even though I was only a few hours old, thanks to Grandpa Walt, my identity was already beginning to be shaped by something that I would *not* be—an invalid. My parents would spend the next 18 years of my life teaching me what I *would* become.

Having been inspired by his father's blunt epiphany, my dad returned to the hospital refreshed and empowered, vowing to treat me like a "normal child." But, even though he probably didn't know it then, he, along with my mom, vowed to do much more that day; instead, they pledged to teach me grit, tenacity, confidence, acceptance, and determination.

-   -   -

After the typical three day stay in the hospital, my parents were finally able to bring me home. Toward evening on the first night, my mom, wanting some alone time, told my dad that she would take me to the nursery to feed me and get me dressed for bed. She kept the room dark, hoping to soothe me so it would be easy to put me to bed. Even before I finished eating, I was fast asleep on her chest. She picked me up and gently set me in the crib. My newborn body was just a speck upon the massive mattress. Crouching down next to the crib, my mom did something that she rarely did. She prayed: "Lord, if you really performed all these miracles that they say you did in the Bible, then you can help Kendra lead a normal life despite her leg, right? If you do, I promise to follow you for the rest of my life."

It might have been more of a conditional plea rather than a prayer, but at that very moment, my mom gave her life to Christ. Although she had been raised in a Christian home, she didn't have a personal relationship with God and was generally skeptical about religion. However, that day she took a leap of faith and gave over the reins, surrendering control that allowed Him to use my birth deformity in accordance to His plans. God used my disability to change the course of her life (which trickled down to my sister and me and now our children). And, it couldn't have come at a better time. My mom needed to lean on her faith to get through the emotional and physical challenges of what was to come.

My parents quickly found out that raising a child with special needs was much more difficult than raising a typical infant. I was not able to take normal baths because of the casts, so my parents had to take a rag and wipe me down with soap and water. Dressing me was also complicated because clothes were hard to fit over my casts and the metal bar. They had to choose outfits that were larger and more flexible than typical infant clothes. Diapers were hard to get around me, so my parents bought them one or two sizes larger to ensure a proper fit. All the newborn outfits and diapers that they were given at the baby shower were bought in vain and promptly put in the donation pile.

When my dad told me about the metal bar as I was in the process of writing this book, I was astounded to hear about it for the first time. Growing up, my parents told me stories of my leg with regularity, so I thought it odd that they would never mention it. Having gained this new information, I inquisitively started sifting through picture albums to see what the bar looked like. However, I couldn't find one single picture where it was visible.

I started to think my dad was making the whole thing up, but after talking about it further, I came to find out that my mom would put me in certain outfits to hide it. She didn't want people to pity me—to look at them with those sad eyes that suggested something was wrong with me. Although my mom knew it wasn't attainable, she hoped that people would have the same blind love and acceptance that my parents had.

I never remember my mom being embarrassed of me and my deformity. However, in those early years, she hadn't quite adjusted yet and didn't know how to deal with the emotional weight of it all. Unfortunately, when they moved past the grieving stage and on to acceptance, I was already too self-absorbed to think about how hard it was for them at the beginning. By the time my memory started to form, they were the encouraging, motivating parents that I remember.

Having that discussion with my dad made the guilt set in. I know that it wouldn't have changed anything, but I wish that I would have been selfless enough to consider it from their perspectives. Raising a newborn is hard enough, but they had to deal with the emotional blow during delivery, the stares, the pity, the questions, the doubt… it was no wonder it took them a little while to adjust to the idea of having a daughter who was "different." Add in taking care of the casts and figuring out how to bathe and dress me to the mix and it quickly surpassed the typical infant care that they had anticipated.

Keeping the casts and bar on for six weeks didn't seem like a long time when the doctors first said it, but near the end, my parents couldn't wait for them to be removed. Not only were they inconvenient, but they reeked! When the doctors at Good Samaritan Hospital finally removed them, my parents were elated.

But, their happiness soon ended when the doctors removed the casts and told my parents that there hadn't been any change to my foot. The cast on my left leg had corrected the dislocation, but that was it. My parents' hope was once again obliterated. The orthopedic surgeon told them that they really only had one option—amputation. My dad, especially, was in disbelief, unwilling to accept that fate.

Upon leaving, they felt hopeless and bitter. "If she's going to be handicapped for the rest of her life, then we're at least going to get some assistance!" my mom told my dad angrily.

They contacted the Ohio Handicapped Association and a couple other organizations, but they were told that they made too much money to qualify for services. The irony of this response is that they were also too poor to do it by themselves. My parents were so upset because they knew the medical costs would be high, and they didn't know how they would even begin to afford it all.

Shortly thereafter, they received a glimmer of hope. When I was about six months old, my dad walked into work at Jack Huelsman's Auto Mall in Fairborn, Ohio. He just so happened to be venting to his co-workers and boss about my condition. He shared his frustrations that all the doctors so far had only given them one option, and he just wasn't willing to accept amputation. That's when my dad's boss, Dick Mannering, told him that he was a Shriner. He explained the partnership that they had with The Shriners Medical Center, a hospital that specializes in limb loss and burn victims. My parents had no idea what a Shriner was, let alone that there was a hospital that was associated with them.

Dick informed my family of all the advantages of being a patient at the Shriners Medical Center located in Lexington, Kentucky:

1. Volunteers from the Shriners Fraternity would come to our house and drive my family the entire way to and from the hospital if we needed/wanted them to. They did this at no charge to the patient's family.

2. If we ever needed to stay the night in Lexington, then we would have help finding accommodations. They partner with the Ronald McDonald house nearby, so, if needed, we could stay there for little to no cost.

3. The proceeds from the Shrine Circus and other fundraising events ensured that whatever my parents' insurance didn't pay, the hospital would fully cover.

Dick planted a seed by informing my parents about the Shriners Medical Center, but when he handed my dad the application, the first thing he saw was a section that asked how much money my parents made and how much they had saved in the bank. Thinking that it was just one more organization that would deny them assistance, they put it aside and dismissed it. Coincidentally, a couple weeks later, one of my dad's long-time customers named Dusty Rhoades came in to get his car serviced.

"Hey, Tim," Dusty said. "I haven't been in since you had your baby. How's everything going?"

"Well, funny you should mention that. She actually had something wrong with her foot when she was born. People are telling us that she might have to have it amputated."

"Oh my gosh, I'm so sorry to hear that. You know there's a hospital that specializes in that in Kentucky, don't ya?"

My dad thought he must be having déjà vu, having just heard practically the same thing from Dick. Was he the only one that didn't know about this elusive hospital? "Yeah, the Shriners Hospitals for Children, right?"

"Oh good, you've heard of it. I'm a part of the Shriners Fraternity that helps out the hospital.

"No shit. Really?"

"Yeah, I guess it's just never come up in conversation, but I've been a part of the group for quite some time."

"My boss just gave me an application a couple weeks ago, but Gail and I make too much money to be accepted. We didn't even fill the damn thing out."

"They aren't really like other organizations," Dusty explained. "They don't care how much you make. They just put that on the application. You should submit it. They'll accept you."

My dad allowed himself to become hopeful despite having been turned down so many times before. "Then, would you do me a favor?" asked my dad.

"What's that?"

"Well, the application said that we need two Shriners to sponsor Kendra. My boss said that he would be one, but would you be the other?"

"Oh, absolutely. I'd be glad to."

Without a second thought (but still thinking it might be too good to be true), my parents filled out the application. Shortly thereafter, I was approved to be seen by their doctors. They wanted to meet me and interview my family to determine if they could provide assistance.

After scheduling an appointment, my parents made the nearly three-hour drive to the hospital from our home in Vandalia, Ohio. With each passing mile, their hope grew.

Upon entering the enormous building, they saw a massive, domed ceiling that had decorative, carousel horses mounted on it. The waiting room had children's toys dispersed all around to entertain the kids. After checking in at the front desk, my parents were given a tour of the hospital. Throughout the tour, they were able to see numerous rooms serving various purposes: imaging, consultation, physical and occupational therapy, surgery, and many more.

The tour guide then briefed my parents on their open-door policy and mission statement. They were shocked to hear about their open-door policy because they thought that it would give the families more privacy with the doors closed. However, the hospital thought it would protect the patients and doctors if nothing could be hidden from the public. At the conclusion of the tour, they heard the PA call out, "Kendra Garman to weigh in please. Kendra Garman to weigh in" in their Southern draw that was completely foreign to us.

Shortly thereafter, we were sent to a room where I would undergo a physical examination and have a consultation with various doctors and clinicians. After enduring the twelve-hour interview process, my parents were completely drained. Although they were antsy to get home after the insanely long day, they were relieved to finally hear options other than amputation.

The people at the Shriners Medical Center explained each choice individually in a way that my parents could easily understand. The options were:

1. I could wear a brace that attached to a special shoe that would hopefully correct the angle of my foot.

2. My foot could be amputated, and I would be fitted for a prosthesis. I would have to receive a new prosthesis roughly every year to eighteen months depending on how much and how often I grew. The Shriners Medical Center's goal would be to provide me

9

with a prosthesis that fit well and met my basic needs. They mentioned to my parents that because they don't require the families to pay for the devices, the legs wouldn't be extravagant by any means, but they would serve their purpose.

3. I could go through numerous leg-lengthening procedures. Each time I grew, the doctors would have to break my bones and then put an external fixator around my leg to stabilize and hold together the broken bones to ensure they grew together in the correct manner. Metal pins or screws would be placed into the bone through small incisions into the skin and muscle. The pins and screws would attach directly to the external fixator. The doctors could then crank on the screws to stretch the surrounding tissue. Although the length discrepancy could only be corrected up to a certain point, they would try their hardest to get my two legs to be the same length. They said that if my parents chose leg lengthening as an option, the doctors would decide later a plan for how to best serve my needs. For example, they could potentially put the screws right into my growth plates to ensure more efficient progress.

4. Bone fusion was also discussed. The surgeons would fuse my ankle to my tibia. However, because of the length discrepancy of approximately an inch and a half, I would still have to wear a shoe with a large platform sole.

Although they were happy to finally have options, none of them seemed to be the perfect fit. Meanwhile, the doctors kindly informed my parents that a decision should be made quickly because, if they chose to amputate, the best option was to do it before I would develop memories and be able to recall the surgery or the fact that I once had a leg. Beyond two years of age, what's known as phantom pains can start to occur. The amputee often has the sensation that their limb is still there. Although, to the layperson, that might seem like an exciting experience, amputees typically characterize the sensation as being very painful, almost like needles being poked into their residual limb.

Eric Miller, the current Manager of Orthotics and Prosthetics at The Shriners Medical Center, said, "Most congenital patients don't experience phantom pain, but it is common in amputees who lose a limb due to trauma. For example, I once had a patient who was involved in an accident. Because of the trauma that she encountered and her age at the time of the accident, she had a very difficult time adjusting, both physically and mentally, to being an amputee. It took her years to come to terms with losing her leg, and it took a very serious psychological toll on her. She was inundated with excruciating phantom pains that made the coping process even more difficult. She told me that it felt like someone was stabbing her with a knife on the bottom of her stump. Certain pressure points on her residual limb would exacerbate the problem when they would come into contact with her socket."

Even though this was the first time my parents had heard of phantom pains, they knew it was something that they wanted to avoid at all costs. Despite all the self-inflicted pressure to make a decision, they still couldn't make up their mind. So, they waited...and waited. When I finally started walking at 18 months, a milestone I reached much later than my peers, they decided to play it safe and went with the least invasive option: a brace. Although doubtful, they hoped with childish fervor that it would be the fix that they were looking for.

However, the brace wasn't effective. One side of the "shoe" was completely worn down from dragging it as I walked, and the angle wasn't corrected in the least. It was another failed attempt.

Valuing their family's opinion, they sought their advice. Everyone pretty much came to the consensus that leg lengthening was not the best option for me. They were concerned about the longevity of the rehabilitation and chronic pain I would likely have to deal with.

About that same time, my parents took my older sister Rachel and me to the Dayton Air Show in the summer of 1986. We loved watching the airplanes and hearing the Vandalia Butler High School Band play. However, as we watched them perform, my parents saw a girl in the band that had a large soled shoe. She seemed to be having minor difficulty executing the formations. They didn't like the look of the shoe and feared that it would limit my mobility. Therefore, they no longer considered bone fusion as an option.

That only left one choice: amputation. But, how could they be the parents that decided to cut off their own daughter's foot? What kind of parents would they be if they did that? What kind would they be if they didn't? They desperately wished they could see into the future in hopes of easing the weight of the decision.

However, even though they were now resigned to the fact that I must lose my foot, they were clueless about what the next steps were. Because my parents were still a little leery about amputation, they decided to have one more consultation with the people at The Shriners Medical Center. On the trip down, they prayed for some sort of sign to tell them what to do or to somehow make the choice easier. Little did they know, they would get their sign that same day.

After a brief stint in the waiting room, we got seated in the brightly colored, animal-themed room and waited patiently for the doctors. Suddenly, someone with a white coat entered the room and shut the door. My parents gave each other a suspicious look because they had been told in their orientation that the hospital had an open-door policy. The abnormally tall, dark-haired man went on to explain that he was a medical resident and then proceeded to do a thorough exam. He stopped abruptly, looked up at my parents and said, "Mr. and Mrs. Garman, the sooner you realize that your daughter has something on the end of her leg that she will never be able to use, the better off you'll be." He shook my parents' hands and briskly walked out of the room.

My parents glanced at each other again, utterly confused. *Where did he go? What did he mean?* They had never encountered a doctor that was so straightforward and adamant on a course of action. Had he really just told them what to do? My parents knew that doctors weren't supposed to do that because it could get them in trouble if something went poorly. The patient might blame the doctor and he/she could end up with a legal matter to deal with.

What made things even more strange was the fact that my parents never saw that man again. That was the first and last time they would meet. A few weeks later, at their next appointment, my dad asked a nurse if he could talk to the resident. She responded with,

"Tim, oddly enough, he only saw one patient during the short stint that he worked here. That patient was your daughter."

To this day, my parents are convinced that the resident was an angel. God had used him to deliver the "sign" that they requested so vehemently. The divine intervention left my parents completely reassured. Instantly, they felt the weight of the decision lifted off their shoulders, leaving them confident that my foot must, in fact, be amputated.

Now that I'm an adult, I can't fathom having to undergo multiple surgeries and endless procedures to still not have full use of my leg. I know it's easy for me to say now that I know how everything played out, but amputation was the only option for me. I'm sure my parents would have loved to be able to consult with the future version of me when they first had to make the decision, but obviously that wasn't an option.

I admire their gumption and bravery. I would be a completely different person if they made a different decision. I can probably even go as far as saying that the outcome wouldn't have been as good.[1]

Now that I have children of my own, I can't imagine giving the doctors my approval to remove one of their limbs. It's counterintuitive; our goal, as parents, is to protect our children, not allow someone to hurt them. Thankfully, however, my parents were able to ignore their natural instinct enough to make the impossible choice.

---

[1] Amputation was right in my particular situation, but in no way am I trying to suggest that it's right for everyone.

13

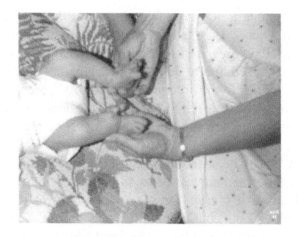

I only had three toes and my ankle joint was malformed. This picture was taken a couple days after my parents brought me home from the hospital.

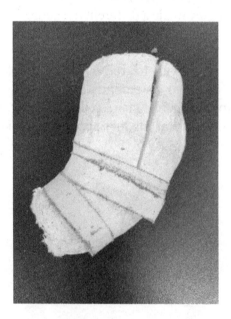

Doctors hoped that by wearing this cast the tendons in my foot would be strengthened, but it didn't work.

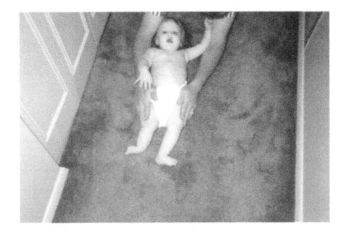

There was about an inch and a half difference in length between my two legs.

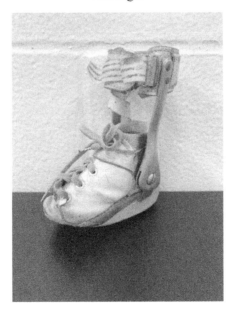

This is the brace that the doctors hoped would straighten the curvature of my foot. However, it made no positive change whatsoever.

Chapter 2

From 8 Toes to 5

At 23 months, I arrived once again at the Shriners Medical Center for my amputation. My parents, sister, aunt Joyce, and grandparents all sat in the waiting room with me while the doctors and nurses prepared for the impending surgery. Everyone was nervous except for me, for ignorance truly was bliss in this scenario. I played with practically all the toys that the hospital had, and my family members took turns pulling me around the hospital in a red wagon to pass the time until I got called back to the surgical room. The only thing that seemed to bother me was the fact that I wasn't allowed to eat or drink anything because of the anesthesia that would be administered during the surgery. Finally, a nurse came out of a set of double doors and called, "Kendra Garman?"

My dad picked me up and carried me over to where she was standing.

"Can everyone come?" my dad asked, trying to sound calm and collected.

"Sure, but only until we get to the operating room doors. You can give her hugs and kisses there, but then you'll need to come back out here and wait until the surgery is over," she explained.

My dad waved to everyone, signaling for them to follow. As we all walked down the hall, it was silent. No one knew what to say. They didn't want to make a big deal out of things for fear of scaring me.

When we reached the door, everyone took their turns holding me and giving me hugs, prolonging the inevitable.

"You're going to be ok, sweetie. We love you very much. We'll see you in just a little bit, ok?" my mom said reassuringly. The nurse held out her arms so that my mom could hand her over. That moment was the hardest part of the process. There was so much trust involved—trust that the amputation was the right decision, trust that the doctors knew what they were doing, and most importantly, trust that nothing would go wrong during surgery.

Even though she wanted to keep holding on, my mom eventually gave me to the nurse.

"She's in good hands. We'll let you know when she's in recovery, ok?" the nurse said.

After the doors closed and they could no longer see me, they retreated to the waiting room. I obviously don't recall any of this day. The whole point of doing it at that precise time was so I *wouldn't* have any memory of it. So, I had to rely on my aunt Joyce, my mom's older sister, to share the events of that day. My dad's memory was a bit spotty because of the emotional gravity of the situation.

I will never forget the day that I received an email from my aunt containing all the specifics. I was sitting in a lawn chair in my driveway on Halloween night with a big bucket of candy on my lap. My husband paraded our daughters around the neighborhood in their adorable costumes. During a lull in the trick-or-treat action, I read through my aunt's reflection. I only got through two paragraphs before I felt the tears streaming down my face. (Thank goodness it was dark or there would have been some confused kids). It wasn't her words on the screen that affected me necessarily, but the overwhelming sense of loss from having to piece together parts of my life from someone other than my own mother. My mom died four years ago, and the memories that I never even thought to ask her when she was alive died with her. Thankfully, I have acquired plenty of information from my other family members, but I still can't help to feel the absence of my mom in this process.

As I read further through the email that night, my aunt Joyce's anecdotes really helped to lighten my mood. For example, she shared that since both she and my mom were stress eaters and had a bit of a sweet tooth, they went through an entire family-size bag of peanut M&M's and another whole bag of plain M&M's while they anxiously waited for the surgery to finish. They were told that the surgery would take approximately two hours. So, when two and a half hours had passed, everyone started becoming anxious.

"Why haven't they come to get us yet?" my mom questioned.

"I have no idea. What do you think is taking so long?" said my dad.

"Do you think something went wrong? They would tell us, right?" My mom was always a worrier. She would fret about the weather, my dad's driving, being late, but in this situation, her anxiety was probably warranted.

"I'm sure they would," my dad reassured her. "Maybe I should go ask someone for an update..."

A woman in the waiting room that was sitting nearby approached them. "I overheard ya'll talking," she began in her Southern accent, "and I saw a bunch of kids in the recovery area. I bet if you go over there, you'll at least be able to ask what's goin' on." She pointed them in the right direction, and my parents immediately left their seats and headed that way, grateful for the woman's help.

When, at last, my parents were allowed into my recovery room, they saw their groggy little girl coming out of anesthesia. I was sitting in a crib with a cast up to mid-thigh. Although they thought they were mentally prepared to see the absence of my foot, it still took a while for it to sink in. My foot was gone. Irretrievably gone. To them, it was a relief to be rid of a part of me that was obviously holding me back, but they couldn't help but feel a sense of loss.

During the surgery, the doctors conducted what was called a Symes Boyd Amputation. The goal of the procedure was to keep as much of my leg as possible and maintain my calcaneus bone, otherwise known as the heel bone, in order to provide stability. They also salvaged the heel pad so that I would have something cushiony to walk on when my prosthesis was off. Additionally, surgeons who perform Symes Boyd amputations tend to leave a round, bulbous distal end to help suspend the prosthesis. Leaving a large, ball-shaped portion at the end of the stump gives the prosthesis something to hold onto.

The ligaments and tendons attaching the foot to the ankle were cut and arteries were tied off and then cut as well. My heel pad was then stitched back on the end of my residual limb. There was an incision that was made on my shin where they performed all the inner portions of the surgery. It left a scar that they called a dimple due to

19

its resemblance to a dimple on someone's cheek. In later years, I would learn to wiggle my stump, draw faces on it, and play games like "catch the stump." But, by no means was the recovery fun and games.

When I saw my parents come into the recovery room, I got excited. I started to stand up, putting my full weight on my newly amputated stump. I was too young to realize that it would be painful, but it didn't take long for me to realize my mistake. I let out the most horrific scream. My parents rushed to the crib to console me. However, they needed as much consoling as I did. It broke their hearts to know that their daughter was in pain and they could do nothing to fix it. They were completely helpless. My parents tried for hours to get the heart-wrenching sound out of their minds. In fact, my mom still spoke of that incident decades after it occurred, speaking volumes to the fact that it was imprinted on her mind indefinitely. I'm sure they wish they could erase their memories of the surgery, but I am selfishly thankful that I have absolutely no recollection of the amputation or its aftermath, nor did I ever experience any phantom pains. I'm forever grateful that my parents not only made the decision that they did but made it *when* they did.

After the doctors got my pain under control and the swelling started to subside, my parents were flabbergasted at the ease with which I was able to stand on my own. At that moment, they were again reassured that they had in fact made the right decision.

Because my parents wanted things to be as "normal" as possible for me during my week's stay in the hospital, they stayed with me each night. Meanwhile, my grandparents brought my sister Rachel to Kentucky, and they stayed in a hotel nearby so they could visit daily. Rachel recalls it being like vacation and not really understanding the gravity of the situation. That was somewhat due to her only being five at the time, but also because no one else in my family made a big deal about it. Rachel reflects that she felt that I was just how I was. It was more of a matter-of-fact situation.

At night, my grandparents and sister would retreat to their hotel room. It was a place of wonder for Rachel. It had a murphy bed, which she had never seen before. She got to sleep in the mystical bed up in a loft all by herself. But, upon waking, my grandparents saw a frightening sight. Rachel had gotten into my grandma's makeup and had painted up her entire face, resembling a clown. Bright pink lipstick was all over her mouth. Blue eye shadow was on her eyelids, but also everywhere else on her face. After their anger subsided, they made light of the situation and took my sister to the hospital without removing the makeup. It was their attempt to make my mom laugh and get her mind off the situation, which inevitably worked of course.

Rachel described my hospital room as being extremely colorful and looking nothing like a hospital. She was almost envious that she didn't get to stay there. It was a testament to how hard the Shriners Medical Center tried to make their patients feel comfortable.

During my week's stay, I was adamant for some reason about getting potty trained. My mom wanted nothing to do with it, believing it would be a much easier process to start in the comfort of our home. But, true to my nature, I was stubborn and demanded going to the potty right then. My mom would stand in the bathroom with me making up silly potty songs like "Tinkle Tinkle Little Star" while I beamed with pride at my success.

At the end of the week, we were finally released from the hospital and were relieved to be home. I had to be in the cast for 6-8 weeks before getting fitted for my first prosthesis. When talking to Eric Miller, he stated that the recovery time is still roughly the same today. However, they now have the patients wear a sleeve over the stump called a shrinker to better aid in the reduction of swelling.

When in the cast, I didn't use a wheelchair or crutches; I hobbled around directly on the cast while I got used to the even larger length difference between my two legs. Since I was a rambunctious toddler, I didn't really have the patience to sit in a wheelchair for any length of time. And, I probably wouldn't have been able to maneuver on crutches since I had only learned to walk a few months prior. But, I didn't really need any of those tools. I quickly became a skilled cast walker and was able to deftly perform my normal tasks.

-    -   -

Finally, the much-anticipated day arrived. It was time to once again go to Kentucky to see if I was ready to get fitted for my first prosthesis. The doctors did a final check to ensure that the swelling had subsided and the wound was fully healed. Thankfully, everything looked good enough to proceed.

My prosthetist, Wayne Cottle, took out some cylindrical bags made out of a foil-like material. He opened the first bag and pulled out the contents: a white bandage roll. Then, he got a bucket and filled it with warm water. He dunked the first bandage roll into the water and told me to extend my stump. He started to wrap it, layer by layer, until it was fairly thick. It was warm and gooey, so just like every other kid that loves all things messy and dirty, I enjoyed the process. Wayne then ran his hands over the outer layer again and again until it was smooth. He explained that we would wait for it to dry and harden, forming a cast. My parents remember the floor, and Wayne's clothes for that matter, being speckled with dots of white, plastery liquid residue and me commenting on how squishy it felt. It was definitely a new process for my family, but I handled it very well and remained calm until…they got out the tool to cut the cast off. After seeing the circular, bladed end, I had it in my mind that it was going to cut through my skin. I urgently retracted my stump and wouldn't let that thing anywhere near me! It wasn't until Wayne turned it on and let the tool run against the palm of his hand that I finally started to calm down. Nothing had happened to his hand and he was still in one piece, so my little two-year-old mind accepted the fact that I would be safe and succumbed to the dreaded tool. After the process was complete, we were once again sent home to wait. Wayne needed time to construct his masterpiece.

After the cast was taken off, I walked on my bare stump for the first time. Due to the now eight-inch length difference of my two legs, it took a good amount of practice to adjust. I would parade around my house hobbling to and fro. However, traveling outside of the house proved to be more challenging. My parents would have to carry me most times, which, for an independent, energy-filled toddler, was an unacceptable means of locomotion. On one occasion, I stepped on a pebble while playing outside and started wailing for my parents, tears streaming down my face.

Needless to say, when the call came from the Shriners Medical Center about three weeks later saying that my prosthesis was ready, we were all ecstatic. During the 1980's, plastics, polycarbonates, resins, and laminates were mostly used to make the socket. Mine was a combination of these materials. It had a rubber foot with no toes. It was just arched where the toes would be. The bottom of the foot had a bolt that connected the foot to the socket. A simple strap attached the artificial leg to my thigh. By current standards, my leg was very rudimentary. Technology would advance rapidly in the coming years, but at that time, my whole family viewed it like Christmas morning. That was the best, cutting edge technology of the time, and we were all so grateful to be getting it free of cost.

Wayne got out bags and bags of thigh-length socks from a drawer. My parents explained to me that they were all different levels of thickness. We conducted this trial and error method of fitting for quite a while. I would try on one arrangement of socks (to cut down on friction), and it would be too thick, causing my leg to fit too tightly and get tingly. Looking back, knowing what I do now about the fitting process, Wayne had to be an extremely patient person. Prosthetists must rely almost solely on the patient to tell them how things feel and where any issues might be occurring. Being two at the time, I imagine that I had a hard time articulating the correct information in a comprehensive way. But, my prosthetist didn't seem to blink an eye. Wayne was experienced and knowledgeable on toddler speak apparently, which is good because I couldn't even say the word "tingly." Instead, I assume I said words like "owie" or simply just pointed to the problem area.

After the socks were finally decided upon, I was told to point to areas that caused me pain on my stump. Wayne then put bright red lipstick on my stump sock and told me to walk around a bit. While walking, the lipstick rubbed off on the inner part of the socket. This helped the technicians to detect the exact location where they should grind down the plastic, allowing for a better fit.

I'm amazed that using lipstick in this manner is still considered best practice. It seems odd that there hasn't been some kind of new technology to determine troublesome areas, but after seeing countless prosthetists, all of them have done it this way.

After all the kinks were worked out, my parents were amazed at how easily and quickly I learned to walk on my artificial limb. After a few hours, I was walking better with my prosthesis than when I walked into the hospital that morning with no leg.

Wayne wanted me to get used to the prosthesis and find other, smaller troublesome areas, so he sent us out to lunch. He knew we lived a good distance away, so any tweaking needed to be done before I was sent home.

We went to our normal restaurant, Shoney's. We didn't have any Shoney's up North, so when we found one near the hospital, it was decided that that would be our new go-to restaurant on our visits. I remember getting to choose a sucker out of a giant bear statue that had a hollowed-out place in its stomach to house all the multi-colored treats. My family didn't go out to eat very often because money was tight. So, going to a restaurant was certainly special. Getting a sucker or a dessert at lunch was an anomaly in the Garman household. Meals were nutritious, multicolored, and dessert was given after dinner in the occasion that all of one's food was eaten. So, Shoney's was something that I anxiously awaited each trip.

After lunch, we walked around for a couple hours visiting some local stores. Upon our return to the hospital, I was able to point to a few places that hurt. What I couldn't articulate to Wayne, he gathered through observing the red marks on my stump. He tweaked the angle of my foot and did a few other alterations. When Wayne was certain everything was correct, he sent us home and told us to call if we had any problems.

Although the adjustment period was brief and easy, I still came across some challenges. Just as people have to break in a new pair of shoes before running marathons, I too had to get my stump used to the new friction that I encountered and some pressure point issues (especially around my knee). The strap chafed my skin a bit, but the calluses that I built up over time certainly helped me gain comfort.

The weight of my prosthesis was foreign to me as well. I would try to ride my big wheel around the neighborhood, but my right leg kept falling from the pedal since my thigh muscles hadn't developed enough yet from having to carry the extra weight. Additionally, I ran into complications because I didn't have any real toes to assist me in gripping the pedals. Big wheels aren't like typical tricycles in that their pedals are out in front instead of straight under the seat. Therefore, the positioning didn't help my foot stay on either. My dad was bound and determined that my prosthesis was not going to hinder me in any way, so he fabricated a strap that he attached to the right petal. He had a proud moment when he saw that it instantly kept my foot in place. After that, my parents couldn't keep me off it. They tried to instill in me that I could do anything that anyone else could do. If, for some reason, my leg truly held me back, we would find a modification of sorts to ensure that I could still do it, just in my own way. It was this mentality that helped me become successful despite my physical impairment.

After all these years, I still have that first leg in a bag that I keep in my house. Because it's so small, the people who I show it to always tell me that it is "so cute." I can't bring myself to throw it away. It is showing its age with the foot beginning to disintegrate, but it is nostalgic in a way that not many other things are. It was literally a part of me for a year or so. It also serves as a reminder of how far I've come in my journey, but also how far innovation and technology have come as well.

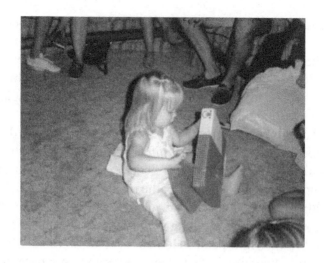

This is a post-amputation picture from when I was two years old. My stump is in the healing process, and I am awaiting my first prosthesis.

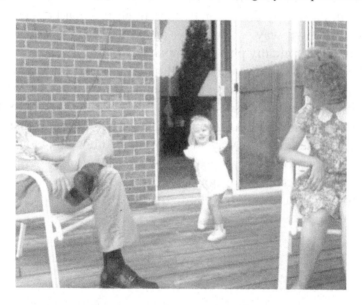

I became a skilled cast walker after surgery. It's still crazy to think about how quickly and easily the human body can adjust.

-My First Prosthesis-

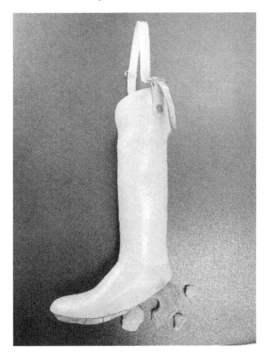

Not that it really held up that great when I wore it, but now that it's 32 years old, it's really in shambles.

Chapter 3

Learning to Laugh

My family's favorite place to go in the summers was Willow Swim Club in Vandalia, Ohio. It was a small pool within walking distance of our neighborhood that had basketball hoops, a volleyball court, a tetherball pole, playhouses, and a concession stand. Because we went there almost every single day, I became very recognizable among the "regulars." It's not hard to miss a girl without her leg on hobbling into the water. My prosthesis wasn't allowed to get wet for fear of it losing some of its durability, so I had to take it off to swim or bathe. Many of the older crowd gave me encouraging glances while the brave ones struck up a conversation with my parents to find out "my story."

However, the kids weren't as tactful and didn't have as much restraint as the adults. One day in particular, my parents were both in the water helping me swim when a group of kids witnessed my prosthesis on top of a lawn chair nearby. They quickly made the connection and figured out that it was mine. They got their goggles on and headed under the water to get a better view of my stump. The kids bobbed up and down for probably five minutes straight and wouldn't stop staring at me. Being about three at the time, I didn't pay much attention to them, but my dad was furious. He hated that I was being made a spectacle of and just wanted them to get lost. But, my mom, a preschool teacher, had a better understanding of young kids. She decided to make it a "teachable moment" as she called it. She asked the kids, "Do you want to know what happened?"

"Yeah!!" they all shouted enthusiastically.

"Well, she was only born with three toes and her foot was crooked, so it was hard for her to walk," she explained.

"Then why does she have that?" one of them asked as he pointed over to my artificial leg.

"Well, the doctors had to remove the bad foot. They gave her that leg so that she would be able to walk better."

"Oh, that's neat," they said in awe.

"Yeah, and she's a lot like you. She can swim too." After she took the time to patiently explain it and put it in a simplistic way that they would understand, they were satisfied and swam off.

She often joked that we should come up with a more exciting story to catch people off guard. "Maybe we should tell people you got bitten by a shark."

"Yeah! Or an alligator," I chimed in.

Although we made light of situations such as the pool incident, my parents were inadvertently trying to teach me how to handle the inevitable question, "What happened to your leg?" all by myself.

When I was roughly four years old, my parents signed me up for swim lessons at that same swim club. They felt it necessary for me to be safe in the water. They were especially concerned with my stamina because I had to exert more energy to stay afloat than other kids.

I arrived at Willow around 9:00 a.m. to begin my lessons each week. Although I liked to swim, I hated the initial plunge into the freezing cold water of the pool. My swim instructor carried around a megaphone and would bark commands at us from the pool deck. Her leathery, orange skin was a testament to the countless hours she spent honing her craft. Even though she was constantly telling me that I swam like a sea horse because my legs were hardly ever on top of the water, her attention to detail helped me to improve immensely. Afterall, she was right; I used my arms for everything and compensated in any way that I could to do the strokes. Although I would never grow up to be an Olympic swimmer by any means, I learned to hold my own in the water and became good enough that my parents felt comfortable letting me swim independently.

Not only did I learn to swim with my leg off, but I also learned how to be active with my leg *on*. My parents witnessed how well I ran and kept up with the other kids while playing in my neighborhood. They didn't want my leg to hold me back from

30

anything, so they decided to sign me up for soccer. Although most parents probably would have been hesitant or worried that I might get hurt or not be able to compete with the other kids, my parents had no such reservations. In fact, they were so happy to prove those doctors wrong who said that I would likely never run. They remember thinking at the time, *If they could see her now...*

However, it really was no fault of those doctors to give such a prognosis. Although I often took for granted how easy running was for me, most other amputees weren't as fortunate. I was one of the only patients at The Shriners Medical Center to attempt such a feat as playing an organized sport. Because of my abnormally long residual limb, I had great range of motion and agility. Wayne was ecstatic to learn that I was going to try to play soccer. Even though I was only five years old, I could tell that he had faith in me and was proud of the obstacle that I was trying to tackle.

The first practice was a bit rocky because I could tell my coach didn't really know how to react. He seemed a bit skeptical of my ability, but as soon as he saw me in action, all his qualms were gone. My teammates asked questions about my leg early on and were curious about what happened. However, once we started playing, it became a non-issue. Because I held my own, there really was nothing else to say on the matter.

Finally, the day that I had anxiously been awaiting came around—my first game. My teammates and I lined up at midfield to get our uniforms checked. Despite the fact that the game hadn't even begun, beads of sweat were already forming on our foreheads due to the heat. My team wore gray jerseys with our team name printed in back letters. Black Umbro shorts and tall, gray socks completed our uniforms. The referee went down the line making sure we had on the right type of cleats, knocked on our shin guards to ensure we had them on, and reminded us to tuck in our shirts if we hadn't already done so. I didn't think much of it when it was my turn because I knew I was dressed properly. However, after knocking on my shin guards, he discovered my prosthesis and said apologetically, "I'm sorry, dear, but I can't let you play with this."

31

I looked at him with wide eyes, not fully understanding what he meant. "Why?" I asked.

"Well, your leg is so hard that it could seriously injure someone. It's just not safe." By this time, my parents, sensing that there was a problem, left their seats in the bleachers and came to my rescue.

"What's the problem, ref?" my dad asked defensively.

The referee repeated what he had told me. My mom placed a hand on my dad's shoulder to calm him down and said, "Look, we definitely don't want anyone to get hurt here, but there has to be some way that she can play. Why doesn't she pull her sock up all the way so that it covers her prosthesis entirely? That will give it some padding so it's not too hard."

His eyes lit up at the suggestion because he, of course, didn't want to tell a child she couldn't play. He quickly gave his consent and the crisis was averted.

Once I started to play, I realized that I could kick the ball a lot further than the other girls because I had a harder foot. My coach put me in the back field and instructed me to boot the ball upfield as hard as I could if the ball came my way. I was thrilled that I could keep up with the other girls and participate in an activity that many of the kids my age took part in. Looking back, I'm sure my coach also put me in that position because it involved the least amount of running (other than the goalie, which at that age, everyone took turns playing).

Everything was going well until, about halfway through the game, the ball started rolling towards me. I remembered what my coach said about kicking it hard and clearing the ball to get it away from our goal. So, I reared back and gave it all I had. My cleat struck the ball, and my leg came forward as I followed through with my kick. However, when my leg was fully extended, I felt my prosthesis loosen. I looked down to see what was wrong, but it was too late. My leg was already flying through the air. Losing balance, I collapsed to the ground. My prosthesis landed in the grass about twenty feet ahead of me.

The referee saw what had occurred and instantly blew his whistle, abruptly stopping the game. I didn't understand why everyone was making such a big deal about it. Initially, I thought it was pretty funny. Afterall, it's not every day you see a flying leg. My prosthesis was habitually falling off at home, so it was nothing new to me. But, as I looked around, the referees started motioning for all the players to sit down on the field and both team's coaches came rushing toward me.

"Kendra, are you ok?" my coach asked, his voice full of concern.

"Yeah, I'm fine. Can you just go get my leg and bring it to me please?" I asked. I looked over and saw my parents making their way over to me, their steps lacking the same urgency as the other adults. They were just as accustomed to my leg falling off as I was and knew there was no real need for concern.

When my coach returned with my leg, the problem became obvious. The strap that went over my knee to hold on the whole prosthesis completely broke off on the interior side. The strap was only being held on by one tiny, silver brad on the other side, leaving it dangling halfway down the prosthesis.

"Do I have to be done playing?" I said.

"No, honey, we'll figure something out," said my dad.

"But how? The strap is broken," I pouted.

"Just relax," my mom said. "Let me think for a second." My mom looked around, trying to figure out a solution. In doing so, she got to survey everyone's reactions. Some people's faces were horrified, some were dumbfounded, while others were sympathetic. Everyone other than my parents just sat or stood there. No one had any idea what to do because it's not every day that they got to witness someone's leg fly off. In a moment of brilliance, my mom walked back to the bleachers.

"Does anyone have a safety pin? Maybe in your purse or something?" she inquired.

Everyone began rummaging through their bags until one lady exclaimed, "I do!"

My mom hurriedly took it from her, as to not delay the game any longer, and safety pinned the two parts of the strap back together where the metal, circular piece that normally connects them had separated and pulled through the cloth-like material.

The game resumed, and I was completely unscathed. If I would have been older, I might have handled it with more embarrassment, but I just wanted to keep playing with my friends. After the game, my parents and I died laughing about it in the car on the way home. What was there to be upset about? I had my rainbow snow cone and snack sized bag of chips (my post-game team snack), I had gotten to play like all the other kids, and I now had a hilarious new story to tell.

- - -

Because my prosthesis was broken, we made an emergency trip to Lexington to have it worked on. Around that time, my parents made a pact to make the three-hour car ride more like a mini-vacation each time we went. They tried everything to make the hospital a positive experience for me. A routine quickly developed where my parents woke Rachel and me up at 6:00 a.m., filled their thermos with coffee, had us pack a bag filled with toys, and then carted us out of the house. My dad always drove on the long trips because my mom hated to drive (especially in the rain). He joked that if Mom was driving, we would never get there because there was no way she would ever go even one mile an hour over the speed limit, and she remained in the right lane at all costs.

My dad pulled into a gas station to fill up, and my sister and I got to go in to the store to pick out whatever goodies we wanted. My breakfast of choice was always a 6-pack of mini chocolate covered doughnuts and a bottle of orange juice. We also loaded our hands full of Twizzlers (at my mom's request), nutty bars, and chips for the return trip. My parents' attempt to make it vacation-like worked without a hitch. We never got to splurge that much on ordinary days, so it was a real treat. I'm sure we had a sugar high for days, but we had a blast.

Rachel and I typically ate our breakfast and tried our hardest to stay awake until we saw the giant clock on the side of the highway in downtown Dayton. But, inevitably, our eyes grew heavy from our early morning wakeup call, and we often didn't meet our goal. When we woke up around Florence Ya'll, a locally prominent inscription which adorns the top of a conspicuous water tower along the I-75 corridor, we would point and scream, "Florence Ya'll" in our twangiest accents. It was a ritual that never seemed to grow old. We would then play games like I Spy or hand-held video games to keep us entertained for the remainder of the trip. As we got into Lexington, my parents would comment on all the exits named after horses, being that the city is known as the horse capital of the world. When we saw the big, green exit sign that said, "Man O' War," we knew we were getting close.

Upon entering the hospital, I saw my friend Hope. I rushed up to her and immediately asked her to play. Hope was someone that I had met a year prior when we were four. We seemed to always cross paths, mostly because all "leg patients" were scheduled for clinic appointments on the same day of the week. She was in a wheelchair and had both of her legs amputated. Hope was blond like me, but a little chubby. Being confined to a wheelchair didn't allow her to move around and burn off extra calories. My parents vaguely remember hearing that she had some kind of disease that attacked her skin. It was eating her flesh at such a rapid pace that amputation was her only option in order to stop it from spreading. At one point, her parents shared that they might have to amputate her hands as well, but it thankfully never got to that point (at least in the time that I knew her).

Hope and I hit it off instantly despite our different personalities. I was more outgoing than she was, but it was so great to have a friend that had a similar life situation. At that point in my life, I only knew of one other person with an artificial leg. Rachel had a friend whose mom was an above the knee amputee and had a very difficult time getting around. She often used a crutch to aid in her walking. However, Hope was my first friend that I directly interacted with that looked like me. She would get out of her wheelchair and play on the floor with me in the waiting room until one of our names was called to go back to weigh in.

Hope, as well as many of the other kids at The Shriners Medical Center, had it worse than me. Everywhere that I turned I saw someone using crutches or a wheelchair. Hardly anyone walked with a gait as smooth and fluid as mine. This might sound arrogant, but it was the truth. It was this same truth that helped me to be grateful for the way I was rather than become resentful or feel sorry for myself. I'm sure it wasn't right to feel pity for all the other patients, but I did. Sometimes I couldn't help but feel a little guilty that I seemed to have it so easy. I wanted all the other patients be able to do what I could but had enough sense at the age of five to understand that that would not be the case.

I never once used the physical and occupational therapy rooms. I didn't need to use any of the assistive tools while in the group play area either. The room was filled with wheelchair ramps and chair rails to hold on to, but I sprinted around the place until I was out of breath. When Wayne wanted me to try out my leg after adjusting it, he put me in between two metal chair rails that were bolted to the floor. Many kids held on to those bars for fear of falling due to lack of stability. However, I remember doing gymnastics moves on them and pulling myself up by my arms and hanging there with my elbows locked.

These realities helped shape my mentality later in life. When people would call me disabled or handicapped, I would have to stifle laughter. I simply didn't believe it. I may not have a foot, but I was certainly not disabled. I was fortunately *able* to do so much. If I hadn't ever met Hope or some of the other kids at the hospital, I might not have appreciated my circumstances as much.

After my brief visit with Hope that day, I walked into one of the patient rooms and waited for Wayne. Not only did he fix my strap, but after doing some measurements, he noticed that I had grown, and my leg was too short. My socket still fit, so instead of having to get fitted for a whole new prosthesis, he was able to attach a wooden extension right at the point where my socket met my foot. He had done this process a couple times before in hopes of saving me the hassle of all the appointments that came with receiving a new prosthesis. By this point, with this being my fourth leg already, I was quite accustomed to the routine.

After handing it back to me, he sat there chuckling, which I got a kick out of because he looked so much like Santa Claus with his long, white beard and husky build. Now he not only looked like Santa, but he sounded the part too.

"What the heck did you do to this thing?" Wayne asked playfully, holding my leg up to me so that I could inspect it.

"What do you mean?" I asked quizzically.

"It's all beat up. Look at how many scratches are on this thing!"

"Oh, yeah," I laughed, "it didn't last more than a week before it got like that."

"Well, we're just gunna have to figure out a better solution for you. We can't have it falling off on the field again. There are new things in the works, but I think the only thing that we can do now is have you wear a soft, mesh brace over top of your leg to keep it from falling off as much. Plus, it will help it from moving up and down and causing you pain."

"That's fine," I told him, innocently trying to reassure him. "The refs will probably like that better anyway since they say my leg it too hard." I had really started to develop a special bond with Wayne. I could tell that he tried everything in his power to keep me comfortable and advocate for me. Because of our age difference, I viewed him like a grandpa of sorts. Wayne was so nurturing and kind, much more than what was expected for someone in his position. He didn't just do his job; making artificial limbs was his calling, his passion.

My parents were always trying to show their gratitude to Wayne. If there was one thing that people knew about Wayne Cottle, it was the fact that he was an avid NASCAR fan. So, my dad would get him all sorts of licensed NASCAR memorabilia. Wayne would always tell my dad that he didn't have to do that, but what he didn't know is that my dad was looking for any tangible way to show appreciation for something that could never quite be fully expressed.

I would like to say that Wayne was able to work miracles and fix my leg indefinitely, but that was not the case. Without new technological advancements, his hands were tied. Therefore, my leg falling off became quite habitual.

- - -

When I was five years old, I started Kindergarten at Helke Elementary School in Vandalia, Ohio. Initially, I struggled academically from being one of the youngest in my class, but I made friends easily and was having a blast.

One day, my teacher called everyone over to sit on the rug for circle time. We were instructed to sit crisscross applesauce, so following suite, I did just that. However, in doing so, my leg strap came unbuckled somehow and the whole prosthesis fell off. My classmates had mixed reactions. Some were frightened while others thought it was cool. I was so used to it at that point that I was unfazed.

My teacher came over to me and asked if I needed help. We both tried to get my prosthesis back on but couldn't figure out how. It sounds easy, but it was difficult to determine which part went where and what hooked to what. My teacher helped me hobble to the nurse's office while they called my mom.

When my mom finally walked into the tiny room, she chuckled and said, "Your leg fell off again, huh?"

"You're not mad?" I asked.

"No, why would I be mad? These are things we can't control, Kendra. Let's just get it on so that I can go back to work." I was relieved that she was handling it so well. The people pleaser in me didn't want to upset or inconvenience her. "Let's go into the bathroom and take your pants off, ok? It'll be easier to get the strap back on that way."

After a few short minutes, I was back to class and my mom was in route to Ginghamsburg Preschool. Somehow, she didn't let her frustration show. Having been a teacher for quite some time, I know how stressful it is to try to find a sub on short notice. She had to be flustered, but that just goes to show the amount of patience she had acquired through years of raising a child with special needs. However, her docility would be tested again just a few short weeks later.

My parents were in a bowling league on Friday nights in Dayton. My sister and I loved it because we got to stay up late and my parents would give us both some change to play arcade games. We got to hang out in one of the back rooms with all the other kids while our parents bowled. Childcare was included in the cost of their league, so they were thrilled to have some adult time.

Everything was going well until my parents heard the following message come over the intercom: "Would the parents of Kendra Garman please come to the front desk."

"Oh jeez. I wonder what happened," my dad said to my mom in a somewhat concerned tone.

"I bet you anything her leg fell off again," she said, not the least bit concerned.

"You think so?" my dad asked.

"I dunno. Just a hunch." She walked quickly up to the counter and started inquiring about me. "You paged for us?"

"Uh, yeah," the young worker who was roughly 20 years old said. My mom could tell he was uncomfortable.

"What's the problem?" she prodded.

"Well, there is a bit of an issue. Would you mind following me to the play area?"

"Sure, but, what kind of problem?" my mom inquired, becoming slightly more nervous.

As they started walking towards the room and they were away from most other patrons, the worker awkwardly stammered, "Well, ma'am, her uh, her leg seems to have, um, fallen off."

My mom started laughing, the anxiety immediately diminishing. "That's all? Man, you had me scared for a second. I told my husband that that's what happened."

The worker was relieved that she handled the information so calmly. "Oh, so it's not a big deal?"

"Not at all. It happens all the time. I'll put it back on really quickly."

My mom peered through the glass window of the wooden door before entering the room and saw me sitting on the carpet with my leg in my hands. The second she sauntered in, she spotted the horrified look on the childcare worker's face.

"I'm so sorry. I had no idea what to do. I tried to put it back on, but her pants kept getting in the way," she frantically explained.

"No, don't worry. It's our fault. We didn't even think to warn you that she was an amputee. Sometimes it slips our mind."

As she had done many times before, she reconnected my prosthesis. The young worker stared in amazement and said, "You make it look so easy."

"Well, you kind of get used to it."

After the show was over, I went right back to playing, and she left with a smile on her face because she got to go back and tell my dad that she'd been right after all.

-5 Years Old-

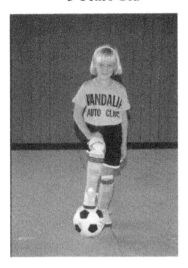

This is the team that I played on when my leg came flying off. I didn't have the sock pulled over my knee for the pictures, but during the game, I had to in order for the referees to let me play.

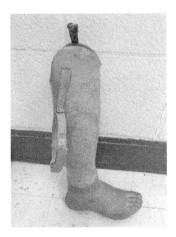

This is the leg that broke in the soccer game when I was 5. Right above my foot is where the extension wedge was placed to add height instead of having to make me a new prosthesis.

Chapter 4

Taking the Suck out of Suction

Although we tried to remain patient throughout all the instances of my leg falling off, there came a point when I was about eight years old when we had had enough. I was due for another prosthesis anyway because I had just gone through a big growth spurt, so we decided to talk to Wayne about other options. Sports had become my favorite pastime. In addition to soccer, I was now playing basketball and softball.

Between all the sports, soccer proved to be the most challenging for me due to the copious amount of running. The strap wasn't only a problem because of how often it would break or fall off, but it was also extremely painful. Because the strap was unable to keep my prosthesis tight against my skin, it would often move up and down on my stump while I ran. Friction was not a friend of mine. Despite the thick socks that I wore under my leg, I was still inundated with blisters and other skin abrasions on a regular basis. The blisters would form mostly around my knee, my dimple, and the area where my heel was stitched on at the bottom of my stump. The continued friction would rub the skin raw and make it peel off. I would put Band-Aids and ointment on, but they caused a different type of discomfort. The bandages weren't smooth, so they were just something else to rub against.

My parents had no idea how I could keep going. They told me I didn't have to play, but I was always determined to fight through it. I never cried because of the pain—ever. I'm not sure if I realized at that young age that crying wouldn't do anything to help the situation, or if I was too prideful to admit that it got to me. My parents, on the other hand, would grimace when I ran because they knew how much pain it was causing me. It was clear to all of us that the strap would no longer suffice. Although I tried to stay strong through the pain, I saw my breaking point in my near future. Something had to change.

Wayne hated to see the limitations that the strap put upon me, so he suggested that I try something different: Semi Suction Suspension. There are many different types of suction legs. Some involve a one-way valve that removes all the air from the leg and restricts any more from entering, thus creating a seal. But, the one that Wayne wanted me to try was only partially held on by suction. I would have an inner sheath that would fit snugly inside of the outer socket. That sheath was made out of a grippy material that wouldn't easily slide in and out. Because my bulbous distal end was thicker than the middle portion of my leg, the socket didn't allow it to lift up into the narrower part of my prosthesis. Patients with longer residual limbs, such as myself, normally find more success than others whose stumps are shorter.

Without even knowing all the details, I was elated. No more strap… that's all I needed to hear. That fact alone was a game changer in my book.

Wayne told me that practically everything else, other than the method of attachment, would be the exact same when compared to my current leg; I would still wear socks underneath and have a foot that would screw into the socket. It would also still be made of the same hard, durable materials. However, Wayne saved the best information for last—my foot would now have toes. Whereas before, my foot was just smooth and arched, now it was going to look more realistic.

"You wanna know something else?" asked Wayne. "We can now add dye to the laminate when making your leg, so you get to choose a color that matches your skin tone." Wayne presented me with about twenty color swatches that were held together with a silver ring. I put each one against my skin to determine the closest possible match. That moment was the first time that it even occurred to me to desire a prosthesis that was realistic. Up to this point, I cared about functionality before aesthetics. Now that I knew it was an option to make my prosthesis look like my real leg, I wanted nothing more than for that to happen (which is an attribute that remains true to this day).

44

"Now, this is only if you don't want a design on your prosthesis," Wayne said. "We just got a special printer that can imbed the ink into the prosthetic material or it can be done as a laminate sleeve. The image would wrap around the whole leg. You can get any image that you want: Disney characters, sports teams…" He held up one of his other patient's leg that contained the Cincinnati Red's logo to show me an example.

It's probably no surprise that I wasn't interested in obtaining a design on my leg. I thought that the designs looked neat and the personalization was a great touch, but I wanted nothing to do with any of the options. They would put me further away from my goal of looking like everyone else. This stands out in my memory as being a pivotal moment: I no longer just wanted to be a kid but started caring about fitting in and looking like a young lady. Before, if my leg could keep up with what I wanted it to do, then I was satisfied. Now, I had higher expectations. I wanted it to look feminine and pretty.

A few weeks later, Wayne was able to get my new leg finished. I couldn't believe how big of a difference there was between the appearance of my old leg versus that of the new. It was like I had jumped ten years into the future. The foot was probably the biggest change that I noted. Not only did it have toes like Wayne assured me it would, but it even had indentations where toenails would be.

I looked up at Wayne with bright eyes. "Can I paint the toe nails?"

He was completely caught off guard. It seemed that no one had ever asked that question, and because he was an older male, the idea of painting prosthetic toes had never crossed his mind. "Uh, I guess so. But, I would test it on a very small spot on the bottom of your foot first to see how the material holds up. You'll have to use nail polish remover to get the paint off, and I'm not sure how that process will go."

I couldn't wait to see how the new leg felt. I took it "out for a test drive" as I liked to call it and immediately started running through the hallways. It fit a lot more snugly, so initially it was a bit painful because of all the pressure. Wayne explained that it had to fit tighter because if it didn't, the leg would lose suction.

Upon returning home, I found the acclimation period was definitely longer than any other transition to a leg with a strap that I'd had up to that point. But, to take my mind off the discomfort, I decided to put my nail polish experiment into action. I applied a small dab of bright pink paint onto the bottom of my foot just like Wayne suggested. I let it dry and waited a few hours. Then, I took a cotton ball with a small amount of nail polish remover on it and wiped off the polish. It worked without any harm being done to the rubber material. So, I giddily gave myself a full pedicure. However, unlike most other people, I took my leg off to get a better angle while painting. I guess that is one advantage that I have over the rest of the population. That was the first time in my entire life that I had matching toe nail polish on both feet. I was feeling more "normal" than ever before.

Once I got through the breaking in period, I saw a vast improvement in my overall comfort and functionality. My leg still fell off on occasion, and it still caused me to have sores, but not nearly as often or as severe as what I encountered with the strap.

With all the positive changes, I quickly saw a drastic improvement in athletics. I could run faster and had more range of motion. That summer, when I was nine years old, I was chosen to be on the all-star team for softball. My coaches were impressed with how hard I could throw the ball and how consistent of a hitter I was. And, even though I was new to basketball, I was one of the better ones on my team. I was easily able to dive after loose balls and jump better for rebounds. The suction prosthesis helped very minimally with soccer; I was now able to keep up with the other girls a little better even though it still didn't come easily.

However, my growing confidence didn't just stop on the field or court, it trickled into all areas of my life. That summer, my family and I went to Willow Swim Club like usual. But, with self-assuredness came bravery. My friends were all taking turns going off the diving board. They were great swimmers because they practically lived at the pool like I did. At the beginning of summer, my parents and Rachel taught me how to dive, and after practicing off the side of the pool for a few weeks, I got the courage to try it off the diving board. After doing it once, I fell in love with the thrill and did it repeatedly.

But, always a step ahead, my friends then started doing front flips off the board. I had done front flips while in the water hundreds of times, but doing it off of the diving board was a different venture altogether. I finally gained enough courage to attempt it. I hobbled up to the diving board- one step with my left knee extended, growing taller, then one step onto my right stump, sinking down eight inches. I repeated that process until I reached the ladder. I knew the cards were stacked against me before I even jumped: I wasn't able to jump on the end of the board like everyone else to get the spring that I needed to complete the task. Without my leg on, I didn't have toes, so I couldn't grip the soaking wet board as easily. And lastly, another problem that I ran into was the eight-inch length difference between my two legs. When I stood on both legs at once, I was much shorter, so I was closer to the water than my friends. For all these reasons, I was concerned about performing an awe-inspiring face smacker in front of everyone at the pool that day.

I must have stood up there for five minutes trying to amass the courage to jump. The number of kids lining up behind me made me all the more anxious.

"Do you want to go ahead of me?" I asked the next girl in line.

"No, it's fine. I can wait," she said politely.

At one point, I looked around and saw a small audience begin to gather. Both adults and kids assembled around the edge of the deep end and shouted their encouragement; even the lifeguards started to join in.

Finally, with all their help, I sprung off the board. I had worked it out in my head that I had to tuck tighter to get the flip finished in time. It wasn't perfect, because I actually over rotated a bit, but I did it! When I came up to the surface, I could hear people clapping and cheering. I couldn't believe they were showing that much support and were interested in a little girl's internal battle of self-doubt. After all, it was just a kid doing a front flip. But, to me, it was so much more than that; it was reassurance that I could do more than I thought I was capable of. Without having learned that, I probably never would have agreed to my next adventure.

- - -

One evening around dinnertime, my parents got a call from the Shriners Fraternity. Many years prior, the Antioch branch in Dayton had sponsored me and helped me get connected to the Shriners Medical Center. But now, they were seeking *my* help.

The man on the other side of the telephone said, "Hi, can I speak to Tim or Gail Garman?"

"Yes, this is Tim," my dad responded.

"Hi, I'm calling from the Shriners Fraternity to ask a favor of Kendra. We have a lot of new members, and we thought that maybe she could tell them about her life as an amputee and her experience with the Shriners Hospital for Children."

"Uh, what exactly would that entail?"

"Well, we want her to come to the Antioch Temple in Dayton and give a speech. We're hoping that after the members hear Kendra's story, they will be more inclined to donate funds and help support the hospital."

"I'll have to talk it over with her, but we've had an amazing experience there, so we'd love to help. If nothing else, I wouldn't mind sharing my perspective."

"That'd be great. Why don't you discuss it with her and then get back with us?" he suggested.

My dad hung up the phone and turned to me. I had been listening in, my curiosity getting the better of me. "They want you to give a speech. What are your thoughts? You don't have to by any means. But, I do think it would be a good way to give back to them for everything they've done for you."

"A speech?" I said hesitantly. "I hate talking in front of people, especially people I don't know!"

"I know. It's pretty intimidating. I'll be right there with you though. I don't like doing it either, but I think we should. You can write it all out on notecards and then just read it to everyone if you think that would make it easier."

"Alright, I guess I'll do it. But, what do I say?"

"Just tell them the truth. That's all they're looking for. Tell them about how you became an amputee, how you get your legs for free, how the doctors work to get your prosthesis to fit so it doesn't hurt... stuff like that," my dad suggested.

Over the next few days, I wrote out my speech on notecards like my dad suggested. I talked my parents and sister into acting like the audience so that I could practice on them; I didn't want to sound like a blubbering idiot up on the stage. I figured the more I practiced, the more confidence I would have when the time came to deliver the speech.

But, I couldn't have been more wrong. Even on our twenty-minute drive down to Dayton, I could feel my heart start to race. I tried to talk to my dad to get my mind off it, which helped a bit. We parked on the street, and I looked out of the window at the Antioch Temple. It was a pretty building that had a lot of stairs leading up to it. All the nerves that I suppressed during the car ride instantly returned when I looked at the building.

"You ready?" my dad asked, interrupting my thoughts.

"I guess so."

"You'll be fine. You're prepared, so just take a deep breath. Remember, they're not here to judge you. They just want to hear your story. They don't care how well you deliver your speech."

"Yeah, I guess you're right." I opened the car door and slowly made my way up the stairs.

When we walked in, there was an older man that greeted us. He seemed to be expecting us and knew who we were without any introductions. He led us into a big conference room that had a bunch of chairs facing a stage. I hoped that the dim lighting of the room would mask my nerves. A lot of older men with funny looking, maroon hats with gold tassels hanging down the side came up and introduced themselves to me. They wore matching maroon blazers embroidered with their fraternity's insignia. The men were all so nice and welcoming, but I only had one thing on my mind—the speech.

"Do you know what those hats are called?" my dad whispered to me when we got a second alone, once again trying to lighten the mood.

"No, what?"

"A fez."

I giggled. "That's a funny name. Why do they wear them?" I asked.

"I dunno. I guess to show that they're a part of the fraternity, but other than that, I have no idea."

Someone came up to the podium and asked everyone to take their seats. My dad and I listened as a few of the members welcomed everyone and thanked people for being there. But then, one of the men announced that it was my turn to get up and share my story. My hands instantly started to shake, and my heart was beating out of my chest. I gave one final look at my dad who whispered, "You got this!"

I walked up to the podium and wiped my sweaty palms on my blue and white floral dress. I laid my lined note cards on the light brown, wooden podium for fear of dropping them out of my shaking hands. When I looked out at the audience, I saw that my view was partially blocked by the podium. That meant that the 75-100 adults, who were mostly male, probably couldn't see anything from my nose down because of my height. I began to read with as much inflection and poise as I could muster. But, when I opened my mouth and uttered the first phrase, I didn't recognize my own voice. It was squeaky and timid, sounding even more juvenile than I already was. My voice quivered from the nerves, but I was able to make it steadier as I got further into my speech. I didn't look up at the audience nearly as many times as I had practiced at home. Meeting their eyes meant intimacy and exposure, neither of which did I want anything to do with.

I don't remember exactly what I even said that day because honestly, I tried so hard to erase it from my memory. I paid no attention to the crowd's reaction towards what I was saying either; all I focused on was getting it over with. Somehow, I got through it, though I was no Martin Luther King Jr. What was on my notecards wasn't nearly as eloquently written and my word choice wasn't of the same caliber, but I conveyed the emotions and facts as well as I could at ten years old. The whole speech began and ended in the matter of four short minutes, despite the fact that it seemed to last an eternity. I was so relieved to be finished, but as I looked up at the conclusion of my speech, I saw the entire audience get up on their feet. They were giving me a standing ovation. I couldn't believe it and truthfully didn't fully understand it. I just told my story, which to me, was pretty ordinary. But, I beamed with pride at having survived my first public speaking experience and ventured off stage.

My dad was up next. He was way more composed than I was. If he was nervous, I couldn't tell in the least. He poignantly told his perspective and then took his seat. He nudged me and whispered in jest, "How's come you got a standing ovation and I didn't?"

"Because I'm that awesome," I responded with a laugh. Now that the stressful situation was over, I loosened up enough to joke back.

We were told that we didn't have to stay for the entire meeting because, after we spoke, they were going to talk about a lot of things that didn't really concern us. So, we got up quietly and started to make our exit. Everyone started clapping again as we walked down the center aisle. Then, a middle-aged woman dressed in a nice, expensive-looking pants suit stopped us and held her hand out for me to shake.

"You did such a great job, dear. Thanks for coming today and letting us hear your story. You're a pretty amazing kid, you know that? A real inspiration to us all."

Blushing, I said a simple "thank you" and continued walking out the double doors.

When we got to our car, my dad said, "Do you know who that woman was?"

"Nope, not at all."

"She's the Mayor of Dayton."

"Oh. I just met the Mayor?"

My experience that day momentarily helped me put aside my feelings of insecurity or stage fright. It felt great to give back to an organization that had helped me in so many ways. Giving that speech put things into perspective. Yes, there were aspects of my life that were difficult or even unpleasant, but maybe my mom was right. What if God did make me like this for a reason? The Mayor had said I was an inspiration. I didn't exactly know what was inspiring, but I started to get a sense that I could use my situation to help people.

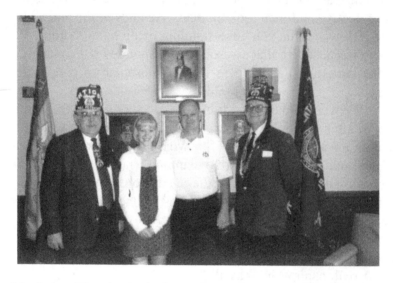

My dad and I at the Antioch Temple in Dayton before I gave my first speech. We are accompanied by two members of the Shriner's Fraternity.

Chapter 5

Suction Sucks After All

Although my suction leg was an improvement over the strap, there came a point, when I was about eleven, that my prosthesis was having trouble keeping up with what the rest of my body was determined to do. Overall, the number of blisters was reduced, but the suction leg still hurt because of how tightly it had to squeeze my stump in order to remain attached. There were days when I could feel my heartbeat in my residual limb. That discomfort was felt in every single step that I took for the duration of the time that I had a suction prosthesis. Thankfully, suction liners are made differently nowadays. Updated technology has proven to be substantially more effective because the amount of pressure isn't needed to keep the leg on.

Not only was the pain difficult to contend with, but the smell became almost intolerable. The inner sheath was thick and absorbent, which created two separate issues. The thickness added to the insulation. When exercising, my leg would sweat, and there would be no way for the heat to escape. And, because it was so absorbent, it soaked up the smell to the point where no matter how many times I washed it, the stench always remained.

Oddly enough, this was the first time that I can remember feeling self-conscious of my leg in any facet. I knew that if I could smell myself, then other people could too. One Friday night, I went over to my best friend Jessi's house for a sleepover with a few other girls. We were all huddled together watching a scary movie and stuffing our faces with an exorbitant amount of junk food when Jessi, who was known for her blunt, tactless delivery at times, loudly said, "Ugh, what stinks? Did someone fart?"

"Oh, it's probably me," I admitted sheepishly. "My leg has really started to smell lately. I've tried everything, but it's just not helping."

"Ew. You really gotta do something about that," Jessi said as she gave me a disgusted look.

"Well, I brought some Quinsana that the hospital gave me. It's this powdery stuff that's supposed to keep my leg dry and make it not stink so bad."

All the girls were interested at that point. They gathered around as I rummaged through my bag to find the white bottle. I took off my leg and shook the powder onto the inner sheath. I then put my prosthesis across the room to air out and be out of smelling range.

My friends certainly didn't have ill intentions. I'm sure they felt comfortable calling me out that way because we were such good friends. Our closeness gave them a pass when it came to keeping it real. I would have been more embarrassed if the harsh words had come from an outsider, but I'd be lying if I said their comments didn't hurt. There was no arguing about it; my prosthesis stunk, but I hated that attention was drawn to it. As I was accustomed to doing, I brushed it off and joined in on the jokes. I thought that if I owned it, then they would have less to "pick at."

-    -   -

In addition to the smell, my foot began to malfunction. That year, I was the backup pitcher on my softball team. I found that there was definitely an art to pitching, and it took a lot of work to refine and hone the technique. I went to numerous pitching clinics and practiced diligently. Despite my efforts, I never quite excelled. I had a lot of speed for my age. In fact, I was probably the fastest pitcher in the league, but accuracy was a different story. On a few occasions, I pitched it over the tall, slanted backstop and the game came to an embarrassing halt until someone in the stands could retrieve the ball.

I didn't just save my wild pitching for the games, though. When I practiced at home, my parents would take turns catching for me. On an especially off day while pitching to my mom, the less athletic parent by far, I threw a ball higher than anticipated. My mom didn't move her glove fast enough, and it hit her right in the face. It seemed like time slowed to a halt as I watched

54

her glasses make the long descent from her face to the concrete sidewalk. I could immediately see the damage that I had caused, although surprisingly enough, it wasn't to the glasses. *They* somehow remained unscathed. My mom's face, on the other hand, wasn't so lucky. The bridge of her nose was swollen and already turning shades of black and blue from where the ball caused her plastic frames to smash into her skin. Needless to say, my mom never caught for me again.

Despite my lack of success, I was determined. If I was having an "on day," I was unstoppable. Girls my age weren't used to my speed, so I struck a lot of people out. My friend Andrea, who was the starting pitcher, would pitch for the first five innings or so, and I would come in to finish the last two.

So, during one of my games, her dad, who was also our head coach, told me that I would be taking the mound the next inning, the top of the sixth. I took my three pre-inning warm up pitches like usual before the catcher yelled, "Coming down!" She threw the ball to second base to simulate a runner stealing a base in order to keep her arm loose.

Then, the umpire called, "Batter up!"

I pitched to the first two batters and quickly struck them out in less than eight total pitches. I set up for the third batter by starting in my normal stance—my right foot on the rubber and my left foot situated about a foot behind. As my arm began the circular wind up, I took a big step with my left leg. In doing so, I had to pivot my right foot a bit to open my hips. (The closing of the hips is what gives the pitcher more force and speed behind the ball). Then, I had to drag my right foot until it was even with my left. If a pitcher didn't drag her foot, then she could get called for crow hopping. If noticed, the umpire could reward the batter first base.

But, as I finished dragging my foot, something didn't feel right. The next thing I knew, I was laying in the freshly-drug dirt on the mound. I looked down to see my foot pointing backwards on my leg.

Despite the fact that I was on the ground, the pitch was close enough to the strike zone that the batter swung. She connected and hit a slow-rolling ball to second base. My teammate threw her out at first. After the play ended, all eyes went to me. My coach ran out of the dugout and motioned for my dad, our assistant coach, to join him. "Somethin' happened to my foot," I said. "Look, it's backwards."

My dad was relieved to hear that it was just an issue with my prosthesis rather than a blown ACL or something more severe. Once the shock of seeing his daughter fall to the ground had worn off, he crouched down to further inspect my leg. He grabbed it in his hand and took off my shoe and sock. After looking at the bottom of my foot, he said, "The screw came loose."

"How'd that happen?" I asked.

"Well, I guess each time you pitch, it loosens ever so slightly when your foot pivots."

"So how do we fix it?" I asked.

"I need an allen wrench."

I let out a groan of frustration, knowing that no one was going to have one of those on hand. It wasn't like the soccer game from when I was five; a simple safety pin wouldn't do the trick this time. I was so mad to have to come out of the game but realized quickly that there was no way that I could just push through it. My coach and my dad helped carry me off the field and sat me down on the bench in our dugout.

Thankfully, one of my teammate's parents, who lived very close to the sports complex, offered to drive my dad back to his house to get an allen wrench. Within 10 minutes, my dad was back and fixed my foot in a matter of seconds. I don't recall if I went back in to pitch that game or not, but you better believe that I was prepared with an entire allen wrench set in my bat bag from that moment on to ensure that same incident didn't occur again. I was probably one of the few seventh-grade girls that knew what an allen wrench was, let alone knew how to use one. But then again, I wasn't the "average" girl.

- - -

When I had to make another trip to Lexington to get my leg repaired, Wayne and I had to have a conversation much like the one we'd had a couple years prior.

"Has anything new come out? This leg just isn't working. I mean, my foot was spinning around in circles during my game the other day, Wayne," I said, exasperated.

"It's funny you mention that. I was going to talk to you about something today. They're trying to design a new foot that would be more responsive and feel like your real one. It's still in the beginning stages, so they are looking for someone who has good mobility that could help them develop a prototype. They said they would pay you for your time. Is that something you would be interested in?"

I looked at my parents to get their take on it. They shrugged, which I took as them letting me have the deciding vote. "Yeah, that sounds awesome!" I exclaimed.

"Ok, I'll get you more information on that, but for the time being, we still need to come up with a solution for your leg breaking so often," Wayne said. "What if I made you another leg?"

"But this one still fits fine," I replied. "You just said nothing new has come out, so what kind would it be?"

"Yeah, I know it still fits, and this one would be exactly like the one you're wearing," he explained.

"Then why give me a second one?" I inquired, not able to make sense of what he was suggesting.

"Well, if you switch back and forth between the two, then you will only wear each one fifty percent of the time. Meaning you'll wear them out half as fast."

It finally clicked. It was a genius suggestion, something that my parents and I would have never thought of.

"Now, before I get your hopes up," Wayne continued, "I need to get permission from the powers that be. I don't think it will go over well. The Shriners Medical Center prides itself on being good stewards of the money that is given to them. They want to make sure we are providing the best care to our patients while still being conscious about overspending. Not only have I never asked to make a second leg for a patient, but to my knowledge, no one else has either. You would be the only patient that has two prostheses."

"We understand it's a long shot," my parents chimed in. "But if you could at least try, we would really appreciate it, Wayne."

He certainly wasn't afraid of pushing the envelope a bit if it meant his patient would benefit in some way. I'm not sure how much coaxing it took, but surprisingly enough, they agreed to his proposal.

So, once again, the fitting process ensued. And, near the end of the day, Wayne was true to his word and got my family more information about me being a test subject.

-   -   -

I didn't really know what to expect when I showed up to the Shriners Medical Center a few weeks later to help them with their new foot design. I was directed to a part of the hospital that I had never been to before. It looked like a physical therapy room. It had a lot of equipment pushed to the side and a big treadmill in the middle. There were lines on the floor made from colorful, electrical tape.

When I got to the room, I was greeted by two biomedical engineers. "Hey, Kendra. Come on in," one of them said. "Why don't you pull up a seat by our computers so that we can explain what we'll be doing today."

Already intrigued by what I saw on their computer screens, I couldn't wait for them to actually start the process. The engineers put little, silver electrodes on every part of me. They used black, electrical tape to affix them to my clothes and shoes.

"We need to put these on you so that we can track your movement. We can watch your gait on our computer and look to see which portions of your foot make contact with the ground. All these things help us determine how to design a foot that would be more responsive."

They had me do every sort of motion imaginable; I walked both slowly and briskly, I ran, did squats, and hopped on one foot. When I was done doing certain movements, they would call me up to their screens so that I could see the computerized version of myself in

58

motion. It was really neat to see everything transferred in this manner. I didn't even know that it was possible to do the things they were doing.

The whole process fascinated me enough to start thinking about a career in prosthetics. I knew the design part wasn't for me. It all seemed over my head, like someone way smarter than me should do it. But, I loved the idea that these people could help so many amputees by designing just one product. Good prosthetists are invaluable, but they can only help the patients that they see. Designing a foot or other prosthetic devices would allow me to help people that I would never even come into contact with. Before that day, I had only considered being a teacher, but I made a point, later in high school, to further research possible careers in the biomedical field. I'm sure that I was slightly swayed by the amount of money that I got for helping them that day. $250 to a 12-year-old was a big deal and was something that stuck with me for some time.

It was many years before I, and many other amputees for that matter, would reap the benefit of that day in the lab. Eventually, their research and creative design helped provide me a top of the line foot that greatly impacted my performance and daily life. That also got me thinking about all the other amputees that have agreed to be a guinea pig of sorts to ensure that the rest of us have quality, comfortable products. It never even crossed my mind to be thankful for those people until I was in that role. I left that day feeling very hopeful that someone out there was going through the same process as me, but instead of testing out a foot, they were testing out a different method of attachment. I remember thinking, *It **has** to be better than suction!*

Chapter 6

Moments of Small-Town Stardom

Most people get their 15 minutes of fame some time or another in their lives. However, I was lucky enough to get a tad bit more than that at an early age. When I was in seventh grade, our neighbor, Ken Palen, approached my parents and asked if he could write an article about me. He was a writer for the *Dayton Daily News* and had observed me playing with his two daughters practically my entire childhood. He was confident that my story would not only catch people's attention and be a good read but would also be inspirational.

My parents agreed without hesitation. They were appreciative to be given a forum to share our story and hopefully help someone in the process. Ken came over to our house with a notebook and a pen, prepared with a dozen or so questions. Most of the questions weren't new to us. Over the years, we'd been asked similar things by people brave enough to break the social code of privacy: "When did you get your foot amputated?" "What is the most difficult thing about being an amputee?" "How often do you have to get a new leg?" After we recited our already rehearsed answers, Ken told us that he would also be interviewing some of my coaches to add more dimension to the article.

I couldn't wait to see it in print. I remember feeling so "cool." I called all my friends and told them that they were going to see me in the paper. I figured it was just going to be a column or two in the back because I knew only the big stories were put in the front and had whole pages devoted to them, but that didn't take away my euphoria.

At the end of the interview, Ken asked my parents for a copy of my softball schedule. He then looked at me and said, "Kendra, I'm going to give one of my coworkers a copy of your schedule so that he can pick a day that works for him to come photograph you in action."

"Is the picture going to be in the paper too?"

"Oh yeah. That's the plan."

"Nice! A photo shoot!" I said jokingly. My parents had to bring me back down out of the clouds after hearing that.

"Now, Kendra, when he comes, you need to just act like he's not even there. Play how you normally would and pay no mind to him, ok?" my mom coached.

"I know, Mom," I said, somewhat annoyed. Like most adolescents, I didn't necessarily want to hear the advice that my mom felt so naturally inclined to give.

When the day came to be photographed at my game, I was even more excited than normal to play. It was perfect softball weather, not blazing hot like during summer league, but not too cold like at the start of the season. My team had on our short sleeve purple jerseys that said "Smith" in gold letters, our matching purple pants, and white, tall socks that had a purple stripe on them.

However, when the game was ready to start and the photographer was nowhere to be found, I started getting disappointed. The game commenced, and I felt deflated, like the wind was taken out of my sail. But after two innings, a disheveled, middle-aged man carrying a black, fancy camera and tripod came walking up to our dugout and started setting up his equipment. A lot of my friends started poking me and pointing. "He's here," one friend whispered.

"I know! But shh... we're gunna get yelled at if we don't focus on the game."

I got my helmet on and pulled a bat out of the rack, preparing for my turn. I went out of the dugout and stood in the on-deck circle. *Act natural. Don't look like an idiot*, I thought to myself. I tried not to think about the photographer, but I secretly hoped I would get a really good hit when he was watching.

When it was finally my turn, I went up to the plate and looked at my coach, who was standing next to third base, to get my sign. His hands moved quickly to make the signal unidentifiable to the other team. I stared intently until I saw the indicator: Coach Sheley's right hand tapping the bill of his hat. Then, his hand swiped from left to right across his waistline, indicating a bunt. With one of my teammates on first and no outs, the sign made sense in order to

62

advance the runner. I wasn't really a power hitter, so bunting became my thing. I was one of the only people on my team that could lay a bunt down consistently. When the pitch came, I pinched the bat with my thumb and first finger behind the thickest part of the aluminum so that my fingers didn't get drilled when I squared up. When the pitcher was halfway through her windup, I positioned the bat so that it was in the strike zone with the bat head higher than the bottom part to help ensure I didn't pop it up. When the ball was close enough to figure out that it was a strike, I made contact and laid the bunt down the third base line. I did as I was taught and didn't look at the ball. Past coaches had impressed upon us that if we did that, it would slow us down, and we would be more likely to be thrown out. Even though I ran as fast as I could, the third baseman had a rocket for an arm and got me out at first. But, I had done my job; I advanced the runner.

After our at bat, my team took the field. I ran out to my position at second base and took some warm up throws to first. When the batter was ready, I shouted encouragement at our pitcher, Andrea. We were best friends from spending so much time together during summer league and school ball. The second hit of the inning came my way—a grounder. I charged the ball and made the short throw to first to get the runner out.

Shortly thereafter, I glanced into the crowd to find the photographer, but I didn't see him. Assuming he got all the shots he needed, I continued playing.

A few days after the photoshoot, the article was published. I remember racing to the end of our driveway to get the newspaper that morning. I ripped the thin, translucent bag off and sprinted inside. I turned to the Lifestyle section where Ken had told us it would be. There I was on the *front* cover. The first two pages of the section were devoted to my story. I couldn't believe the enormous pictures and lengthy article. I certainly wasn't expecting anything that elaborate.

Over the next few days, my parents got many calls from friends and family expressing their support and excitement over the article. I got positive feedback as well. As I was walking through the halls of Smith Middle School, my principal stopped me on my way to class. He told me that he had read the article and was so glad that my story could be an inspiration to others. There was that word again… inspiration.

I was obviously proud of the article, but what I liked most about it was reading the quotes from my coaches. I had never heard them say the things that they did in the article and found it endearing. My softball coach, Rick Sheley, said: "She has terrific lateral movement. She's my starting second baseman and backup catcher…that's a nice accomplishment for a seventh-grader. She's my most aggressive base runner. She's fearless." My volleyball coach, Nicole Burley, said: "I had no idea until the first time she lowered her knee pads in practice and I saw (the prosthesis). Kendra is a very good athlete who became a fine volleyball player for us this year. She moved up to our eighth-grade team for the (postseason) tournament."

I would like to say that my coaches' thoughts of me were all positive, but that wasn't the case. Thankfully, they refrained from publicly sharing my negative traits in the newspaper. Even though they were impressed with my ability and proud of my accomplishments despite my physical limitations, they were less enthralled with my personality. My fiery spirit and stubbornness often had the adverse effect on them. I'm sure it was partially due to my age (the awkward teen years aren't kind to many), but all excuses aside, I was difficult to manage at times. I didn't know how to reign in my stubbornness and only use it for good. Instead, I was just bullheaded in all aspects of my life. I also had a mean streak that I developed as a sort of coping mechanism for the hurtfulness that I had begun to experience from my peers.

When I was in eighth grade, I asked Mr. Sheley to write my senior letter. It, along with the others that people wrote for me, went into a vault of sorts and were given to us when we were seniors. In the early stages of writing this book, when interviews and research were at their peak, I discovered the letter that he wrote me many years prior in an old, white shirt box in my basement. In it, he said, "I remember you as a Dr. Jekyll and Mr. Hyde. Meaning, one day I thought you were a pretty nice kid. You know, pleasant, cooperative, and coachable. The next day you were a real pain in the butt:

64

argumentative, being mean to the other girls, a real brat. I'm sure you're more mature now and that nasty side of you has passed you by. But you're still probably stubborn as all get out. That's ok, nothing wrong with being stubborn." I'm sure I took it as a slap in the face when I was a senior and read it for the first time. However, now that I read it as an adult, I admire his frankness and honesty. I didn't want to believe that I had those qualities, but they are as much a part of me as my prosthesis.

-   -   -

There was a lull in my stardom for about three years until the day that I got the call asking me to throw out the first pitch at the Dayton Dragons baseball game. The Dayton Dragons are a feeder team for the Cincinnati Reds and play their games at Fifth Third Stadium in Dayton, Ohio. The Dragons often chose different organizations to feature at their games, and the Shriners Fraternity just so happened to be who they selected for that one. The Shriners Fraternity also wanted to know if they could interview me a few days prior to the game so that they could write an article to put in their newspaper. Over the span of three years, I had given approximately ten speeches for the organization. Because of my continued involvement, I was an obvious choice to do the honorary task of throwing out the first pitch. I was told that a couple other kids who were treated at the hospital and lived in the Dayton area would be there too.

Three days before the big game, my parents and I went to the Antioch Temple on a Saturday afternoon in order to participate in the interview. Rachel was away at college at the University of Toledo, so it was just the three of us at the time. We were directed to their meeting room, and I sat down on an old, formal looking, floral couch, and my parents sat across from me in separate, leather arm chairs. A photographer took pictures of me as I started to answer the questions that R. E. Beitzel, M.D., the man who was writing the article, was asking me. I wasn't nearly as nervous as I was during my first interview experience. Maybe it was the fact that it wasn't my first time being interviewed, or maybe it was because I was now a sophomore in high school and had matured a bit.

After the article was written and published, the Shriners Fraternity sent me a copy. Above the article was a banner that read, "Shriners Help Kids." The title of the article was, "A Young Lady's Brave Story." Although the title didn't exactly say the word "inspiration," it was conveying the same message to its readers that many people in my life had expressed in the past. By this point, as I became older and more self-aware, I was seriously starting to doubt those types of descriptors. Brave? How was I brave? I considered people to be brave who were afraid of something, but despite their fear, chose to still move forward. Or, maybe they did something extraordinary or heroic. I was none of those things. I just went about living my life and didn't know any different. Being an amputee was part of my identity. Sure, I had struggles (both mentally and physically), but who doesn't? Calling me things like "brave" and "inspirational" just made me feel like an imposter. It set the bar high and the title seemed unattainable. I say this not to appear modest, but to state the truth. Living a life with a prosthesis doesn't make someone inspirational, special, or brave. But, I would later discover that your mentality, who you can help, or the ways that you can give back to society are things that could earn you that designation.

I still have the article, along with some of my other accolades, in the same box of memorabilia as I kept the previous article written when I was in seventh grade. I held onto it to see where I started, and more importantly, where my journey has (and still is) taking me.

Although seeing the article in publication was exciting, I was much more anticipatory of the Dayton Dragons game. I practiced pitching overhand to my dad a few days before the game. I obviously had a lot of softball experience, but pitching overhand was something that I'd never tried. I figured it would be similar to a normal overhand throw, but I wanted to make sure that I actually got it to the catcher and didn't look like a moron.

When the day of the game finally arrived, I remember wanting to wear a Dragons t-shirt, but knew I didn't own anything with their team name on it. So, I had to settle with just wearing their colors—

green and white. My mom, who always swore we were going to be late for everything and would shout, "We're leaving in ten minutes regardless of who is in that car," made my family leave even earlier than necessary to get there on time. Only on this occasion, I knew there was no way they could leave without me since I was the guest of honor.

When we got to the field, we met up with the Entertainment and Game Day Staff. One of the staff members led my family and I to their community room to tell us what to expect. The Shriners Potentate was there to represent the fraternity. My parents informed me that a Potentate had to be elected and it was one of the highest, if not the highest, positions in the fraternity. His head was adorned with the typical maroon fez, and he walked with a cadence that reflected his importance. Dusty Rhoades, one of the two men that sponsored me from the very beginning, was also there for moral support. Two or three other kids, who attended the Shriners Medical Center, and their families were in there as well. I noticed that the kids all seemed to share my nervous energy.

One of the workers got a call on her walkie talkie saying that it was time for us to go on the field. The time had finally come. We lined up and walked in a cluster to one of the entrances that led onto the field. Another organization was being recognized before the Shriners Fraternity, so we waited patiently for our turn. When I looked out onto the field, I saw that members from that organization were throwing out the first pitch too. I was disappointed that I had to share the limelight with so many other people. Like most teenagers, I thought the world revolved around me. When I was told that I would be "throwing out the first pitch," I thought it was more literal than that. Instead, my throw was in fact the sixth or seventh "first" pitch.

However, one of the men from the other organization was quickly able to get me out of my jealous funk by throwing his pitch directly into the dirt. It landed about 10 feet in front of the plate. I tried to stifle my laughter, knowing that it was impolite. After seeing that comical spectacle, I wasn't so worried about my performance anymore. The older man had taken the pressure off everyone else in line, and there was an unspoken air of relief among us all.

When it was my turn, the event staff handed me the baseball and pointed me in the direction of the mound. The ball felt so tiny in my hand since I was used to throwing a softball. I immediately grew nervous because it dawned on me that all my practicing had been in vain. I didn't even own a baseball, nor had I ever thrown one. I hoped that it wouldn't make that much of a difference when it came time to throw it to the catcher. As I started to take my first step onto the field, I heard my name announced over the loudspeaker for everyone in the stadium to hear:

"Making her way onto the field is Kendra Garman. Kendra is a sophomore softball player for the Vandalia Butler Aviators. She has attended the Shriner's Hospital for Children for practically her whole life after being born with a birth defect. She is now an amputee and wears a prosthesis."

When the brief bio concluded, I quickly tried to figure out how to grip the ball. Normally I would put all five fingers around a softball; however, holding the baseball that way didn't feel right. I decided to leave my pinky off so my fingers weren't so crowded. I got into my stance, looked at my target, and hurled it towards the plate. I was thrilled to see that the ball got all the way to the catcher, albeit a little low and not exactly a strike. But, I didn't care; it made it.

After throwing the pitch, I returned to the third base side of the field where Dusty and my parents were waiting. I was still riding the high of throwing the pitch, so when the event staff told my family that we could stay for the game and didn't have to pay for tickets, I was even more excited. We had a great family day filled with eating hot dogs and peanuts, drinking pop, watching the between inning entertainment, and cheering on the Dragons. At one point in the game, my dad leaned over to me and said, "I'm proud of you." Even though I was fifteen, I realized that their pride extended way past the fact that I threw a stupid ball to a glove that day.

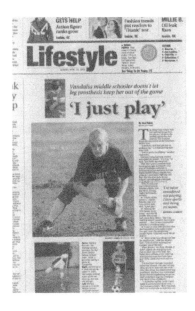

The *Dayton Daily News* article that was written when I was in the 7th grade.

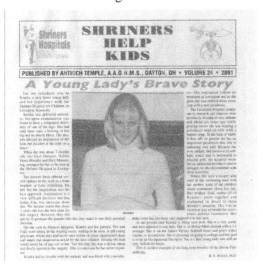

The Shriners Fraternity article written when I was a sophomore in high school.

Chapter 7

The Emotional Toll

I wish I could say that my childhood was filled with being in the spotlight and fun, ego-stroking moments, but that obviously wasn't the case. When the excitement had worn off, I had to deal with the reality that middle schoolers are mean, moody, and emotional. Typically, they lack confidence and they go through a great balancing act in order to find their identity. My experience was no different. My peers were ruthless and self-focused, and I am not naive enough to believe I was any different. Middle school was the first time that I remember being bullied because of my leg, and it took an emotional toll. If I hadn't dealt with the bullying, then maybe I wouldn't have exhibited the traits that my coach, Mr. Sheley, saw. Or, who knows, maybe they're innate personality traits that I would have had regardless of my situation.

One day in seventh grade, I was putting my belongings into my locker as I did between every period. I could feel people watching me, so I quickly glanced over my shoulder. Three boys who I barely knew were standing on the other side of the hallway gawking at me. They were all much shorter than me, seeing that middle school boys tend to physically mature (and I would argue emotionally as well) later than girls.

"Hey, look at that girl's leg," the mousy-looking one said to the others while pointing rudely in my direction. He made no attempt to remain unheard, but instead purposefully broadcasted it for all to hear.

All three boys stopped and stared at me. "It looks like a peg leg," chuckled another.

"Haha. Yeah, just like a pirate!"

Knowing that they were obviously talking about me, I turned around and looked at them so that they knew I heard them. I thought that would stifle their comments, but the exact opposite ended up happening. They then felt called to address me directly.

"I like your peg leg. Will you say ARRG for us? Ya know, like a pirate?" As he said ARRG, his voice cracked ever so slightly.

"What are you talking about. It's called a prosthesis, you know," I retorted forcibly, trying not to show how hurt I was by their comments.

"Whatever. It doesn't matter what it's called. It still looks like a peg leg."

I gave them a death glare, slammed my locker shut, and walked away.

Later, I vented to my friends about the encounter. I was dumbfounded that anyone would be so terse. Because nobody had ever been so outwardly rude, I wasn't really prepared with a comeback. I scolded myself for letting them get the last word and vowed that I would be ready for the next occasion.

My friends took it upon themselves to bravely confront the three boys in a heated three on three discussion in the hallway a few periods later. I wasn't even present at the time. I certainly didn't ask them to stand up for me or accost them, but they felt called to right the wrong for reasons unbeknownst to me. It was almost like the boys had offended them personally.

Despite my friends' attempt to remedy the situation, I remember the boys being unscathed by the encounter. They certainly never apologized. Although their words wounded me to my core, the silver lining was that I had friends in my corner that had my back.

Even though my friends' actions meant the world to me and I knew they were just a bunch of stupid boys, I couldn't seem to shake what they had said. I was much more hurt and embarrassed than angry. Most teenage girls would probably admit that they seek attention from boys and want to be considered attractive. This event somehow seemed to make me question whether or not boys would view me in this way. I didn't want them to see my leg as unattractive or unsightly. More importantly, I didn't want them to deem *me* as unattractive just because of my leg. I didn't realize that the two might be connected until my interaction with them.

When I got off the bus after school that day, my mom was already home from her part-time job. She was able to notice right away that something was wrong.

"What's the matter, Pooh?" (Pooh was a nickname that I acquired much earlier in my life from my love of all things Winnie the Pooh).

"Nothing," I said, trying to treat it like a non-issue.

"Well, I can see something is wrong. If you want to talk about it, I'm here."

No matter how hard I tried, I couldn't restrain the tears that began to well up in my eyes. Those who know me well know that if people coddle me when I'm upset, the floodgates immediately open. Unable to act like nothing was wrong any longer, I cried, "I just wish I never had this leg!" I hated looking weak and admitting that I had let the boys get the better of me, so I ran to my room, shut the door, and continued to sob. My mom gave me some time alone to "get it all out." When she could tell that I had started to calm down, she came into my room to talk about what happened in more depth. I don't recall the exact conversation, but I know she reassured me, told me that boys were stupid, and said that some people just don't know how to react because it's not something that they see very often.

Thankfully, that was the only time my parents or I remember me being so openly resentful of my leg. I'm not sure what it was about that exact situation that affected me so greatly, but it certainly left its emotional scar.

In fact, it affected me so much that I started doing everything in my power to climb the social ladder at school. I thought that if I became popular, it would prove to me and everyone else that I was "normal."

Valerie Stanforth was the most popular girl in the seventh grade. So, what did I do? I sought her out. I started inviting her over to my house to play and quickly became her best friend. Because we looked a lot alike with our straight, blonde hair, our classmates called us twins. Within no time, I had attained my goal. I was now the second most popular girl in my grade.

Unfortunately, that title went to my head. I started being mean to the other girls and abusing my position. If you ever want to know a school's social dynamics, be a fly on the wall in the cafeteria. It will tell you all you need to know. At Smith Middle School, there was a "popular table" where seven of my friends all gathered around to eat. When someone other than our group wanted to sit with us, Valerie and I would make some snide remark and tell them that they had to go somewhere else. We didn't try to hide the fact that they were not wanted.

I'm ashamed of how I treated my classmates, but it just goes to show the lengths that I took to be accepted by others and mask my insecurities.

-   -   -

A few months after the situation at my locker, a similar incident occurred. However, because of my newfound popularity, I handled it much differently. As was the case most Friday nights in the Fall, my family went to the Vandalia Butler High School football game. No one other than my dad was really into the sport, but us girls loved the social aspect of attending each Friday night. All the middle school students sat in the far-right section of the bleachers. Rachel hung out in the high school section that was on the same side of the field but all the way to the left.

My friends and I were just minding our own business and doing our usual—talking about boys and gossiping. Another group of girls were sitting close to us and must have been listening in. I recognized most of them and knew they were all eighth graders. I only knew one of them by name, which was their ringleader, Miranda. She was one of the most popular girls in her grade, had thick, long, chestnut brown hair, and a very mature body for her age. Everyone wanted to look like her, but no one wanted to *be* her. The girls either hated her because they were jealous or because she was a hateful, arrogant piece of work. The few girl friends that she did have clung to her side in hopes of advancing their social status. I can't imagine that they actually enjoyed her company. But, what she lacked in girl friends, she made up for with guys. They flocked to her and were more than willing to give her all the attention that she so desperately craved.

"Did I hear right? You're talking to David?" Miranda asked, rudely butting into our conversation.

"Yeah, we're not official yet though." My body language and tone were definitely dismissive, but of course she didn't drop it that easily. "Why don't you try to date someone in your own grade?"

"What does it matter? He's only one year older than me," I challenged, not knowing why she chose this exact moment to start caring about the inner workings of my life.

"Look, you just stick to your grade and we'll stick to ours. I don't know what he wants with a one-legged whore anyways." She turned back to her cronies who were used to her behavior and said, "Come on. Let's get outta here." They obediently obliged, not straying too far from her heels as they made the descent down the bleachers.

"Do you even know what a whore means?" one of my friends called after her. "Because since she's my best friend, I know she hasn't slept with anyone, let alone a lot of different guys, so you might want to look that word up before using it again."

After she was out of sight, I told my friends that I was going to go tell my sister what had just happened. Jamie volunteered to go with me because our sisters were friends, so we started climbing all the stairs to get to the back of the high school student section. It was intimidating having all the older kids look at us on our way up, so I just tried to keep my eyes faced down so that I wouldn't trip over one of the steps and look like an even bigger idiot. As I got closer to the sophomores, a few of our sisters' friends started saying hi and waving, which helped. In fact, some of the boys in my sister's grade started catcalling and telling Rachel, "Your sister is so hot!" She hated when they said stuff like that. They did it to get a rise out of her, and it worked.

In an attempt to ignore the boys around her and show them that she wasn't fazed by their comments, she turned to me and said, "Hey, what are you doing up here?"

75

"You will never believe what just happened! This girl just called me a one-legged whore."

"Wait, what? What brought this on?" I clued her in on the events that just took place; meanwhile, I could see the protective, older sister side of her start to come out as I finished the story.

"I can't believe she said that to you. I bet she's just jealous."

"Jealous of me... yeah right. You heard me tell you that this is *Miranda*, didn't you?"

"No, I'm serious," Rachel said. "I bet she didn't have an eighth-grade boyfriend when she was a seventh grader. Plus, you're hot."

I rolled my eyes and shrugged off her comment as fiction. I felt at the time that people wouldn't consider me ugly, but it was so hard to feel pretty when my body was going through all sorts of changes. My hair was greasy, I had developed breasts earlier than most, and I started to get a few pimples on my face. People tend to be their own worst critic, and I certainly didn't differ from that norm.

"Well, show me where she is," Rachel said.

"Wait, why?"

"Oh, don't think someone's going to say that about my sister and get away with it. I'm going over there and confronting her."

"Are you serious? I was just venting, but that's awesome. Come on, we'll show you." Jamie's sister tagged along too, not wanting to miss the show and trying to be there for moral support.

The four of us attempted to dodge the crowd and called out our fair share of "excuse me's" as we parted the sea of fans standing alongside the fence. When we got close to the middle school section, we pointed out Miranda so that Rachel could see who she was. She, along with two of her other friends, were standing in the front row of the bleachers leaning their backs against the railing while turned in the opposite direction of the game. That location was pretty typical of the group because they could command so much attention from being in front of the crowd. No one could watch the game without first seeing them.

Rachel, who was normally pretty passive, stood in front of Miranda with more confidence than I had ever seen. She opened off her interrogation by asking, "What'd you say to my sister?"

"I don't know what you're talking about," Miranda answered quickly.

"Oh, but I think you do. Maybe you remember saying one-legged whore? Does that ring a bell?" My sister edged closer to her, almost pinning her to the railing. Jamie and I stared in amazement. My sister had snapped at little kids when they made a rude comment about my leg or when they stared too long, but never had she exhibited this forceful of behavior towards someone. I really thought for a minute that she was going to hit her. Miranda seemed as shocked as we were because no one ever seemed to stand up to her. But somehow, Rachel was able to make her become speechless.

"Well, if I ever hear you say anything about my sister again, we're going to have a problem. Do you understand?"

"Yeah, whatever," she said in her normal tone filled with attitude. But, even though Miranda technically got the last word, Rachel had clearly made her point. In fact, Miranda never once bothered me or even talked to me again for that matter.

When we turned our backs and got out of earshot, I looked at Rachel and said, "That was *so* cool! Did you see her start backing up when you said that? She was actually scared of you. I can't believe it. Thanks so much!"

"Anytime," she said. It was obvious that she was proud of herself too. Although it was uncharacteristic of her to act in that way, it was nice to know that she would do anything to stand up for me and protect me if she needed to. No matter how many sweatshirts of hers that I accidently put holes in, how much I hogged the phone, or how much I begged to tag along with her friends, all of that didn't matter when it really came down to it. She had my back.

- - -

I wish I could say that my personality was the only thing that was impacted from having my foot amputated. However, if I'm being honest with myself, I did much more than alter my personality to deal with the emotional impact that it had on me. I often tried to overcompensate for my leg by making other things about myself appear better or more attractive. I wore too much makeup, I had too many boyfriends, I had my first kiss and mildly "experimented" with boys sooner than my friends and didn't dress modestly to say the least.

I vividly remember walking down the stairs at my house in seventh grade wearing a black tube top that showed my midriff. My friend and I had bought matching ones with our own money and were excited to be going to one of our first boy/girl parties wearing our new purchases. When I got down to the landing, my dad took one look at me and said, "Go change. Now!"

"But, I bought it with my own money!" I protested.

"Yeah, I know, because I would have never bought that for you! You might as well put that in the donation bin because as long as you're under my roof, you're never wearing that." I stomped up the stairs, making a point to let him know that his decision pissed me off.

Similarly, when I was in eighth grade, my dad was doing laundry and found a thong. He asked my sister and I about it, and I admitted that it was mine. He tried to make a joke about it, but I could tell he disapproved and was embarrassed. He said, "What is this slingshot doing in the laundry?"

"Daaad! Give me that! It helps people to not see my underwear lines through my pants."

"You think people are staring at your butt that close?" he asked.

"I don't know! But really, lemme have it. I'll do the laundry," I said.

"Well, I guess I can't argue with that. If it gets me outta doin' the laundry, then that's a win I guess."

Do I wish I would have combatted the hurtful comments and my own insecurities in a healthier manner? Of course, but that just wasn't the case. The internal struggle and self-talk that took place in my mind was all I could do some days to survive the difficulties of becoming a teenager.

Take the pool for example—instead of it being the joyful, easy going atmosphere that I remembered as I kid, it became a place of embarrassment. When the hot guys from my school came to the pool, I wanted to hide. I would do everything I could to get to Willow Swim Club early so that they didn't have to see me take my leg off and get into the pool. My leg was much more hidden when I was already in the water when everyone else arrived. Or, on days where I didn't feel up to dealing with the emotional rollercoaster, I just simply avoided the water entirely. I would be dripping sweat, but I would tell my friends that I wanted to work on my tan. I wanted more than anything to get into the water to cool me down. I hated laying there by myself while all my friends were in the water, but sometimes it just wasn't worth it.

But, on the days that I did get in the water, I dreaded the moment when the lifeguards blew their whistles to signal a rest break. That meant my cover was blown.

I would hobble over to my lawn chair that was turned to face the sun for optimal tanning purposes as quickly as possible and immediately wrap myself in my towel. I slyly dried off my stump while keeping it concealed the entire time. Then, I put my prosthesis on as fast as humanly possible.

The boys never mentioned my leg, so it's not like they were rude or even immature about it. They did absolutely nothing to warrant the type of response that I exhibited. It was all a fabrication of my mind. I somehow convinced myself that they would hold it against me or not view me the same as the other girls.

When rummaging through some old poetry that I wrote during the time, I found this poem that speaks directly to those summer days:

Hidden

Spring fades away and takes
with it my confidence

79

While summer haughtily strolls
in alongside my insecurity

Warmer weather does little
to conceal my deformity
I can no longer hide,
left completely exposed

My difference is accentuated
A spectacle for all to see
A rare treasure put on display
Broadcasted to the masses

I desperately try
to divert their attention
Cover it, disguise it
No one will tell…

But who am I kidding?
Their eyes still see,
Affixed to my aberration
Or a construct of my imagination?

     I certainly didn't have to reread that poem to remember the internal battle that I went through during middle school. It is still crystal clear in my memory. Most people don't have to go through their lives with people blatantly gaping at them. I did. I knew when I took my leg off at that pool, all eyes were on me. When I walked into a store with shorts on, all eyes were on me. When I walked through the hallways at school, all eyes were on me. That has a way of messing with your psyche. It's like their eyes could penetrate through me, leaving me utterly exposed and insecure. Their stares somehow convinced me that something was wrong with me, even though I had been told differently my entire life. The little confidence that I did have was obliterated.

To cope, I started to develop different behaviors to subconsciously cover up and draw less attention to my flaws. When sitting down, I would cross my left leg over my right in order to cover my knee, which was the unsightliest part of my leg. People would often ask me, "What's wrong with your knee?" They would be confused when I told them about my foot being amputated because they wouldn't notice anything other than my knee upon first glance.

Because the outer socket was flesh colored, it matched my other leg fairly closely. Some people couldn't tell that it was a prosthesis until they got close or scrutinized it carefully. However, my white socks that stuck out the top of my prosthesis stood out like a sore thumb. To combat that, I asked Wayne for flesh colored socks. Again, it wasn't anything that he'd ever been asked, so he had to do some investigating. It turned out that he was able to order a very thin, skin-toned sock that I could wear over my white socks. It did wonders in masking my impairment.

Even still, I found myself wearing pants more often than shorts because my prosthesis was completely disguised that way. So many people over the years have told me, "I had no idea you even had a prosthetic leg until I saw you wearing shorts one day. You would never even know. You do so well with it." Pants helped me blend in and have a sense of normalcy. However, no matter how hard I tried to mask it or think up stupid coping mechanisms, nothing could negate the fact that I was *different*.

Chapter 8

Adjusting to High School

Finally, the horrors of middle school ended, and with it, went the hurtful comments. But instead of having to deal with the emotional issues that adolescence presented, I was faced with other types of challenges.

Before my freshman year of high school, I signed up to take my gym class in the summer. I chose this option for many reasons: I wouldn't have to deal with changing clothes and getting sweaty during the school year, I could get the credit out of the way and have room in my schedule to take other classes, and the activities were way more entertaining than during the school year since they offered biking, dancing, canoeing, etc...

Many of my friends decided to take summer gym as well, so we had a blast together every morning for six weeks. I never had trouble doing any of the tasks except for when it came time to canoe. The week before we were set to go, I started mapping out the logistics in my mind. I had been in a canoe before when I was at church camp, but that was just in a circular pond. Because my leg wasn't allowed to get wet, I had taken my leg off and had someone help me get in the canoe. When I was finished paddling around the pond, I got out right at the same place that I got in to retrieve my leg.

But, I knew this canoeing trip would be different. We were expected to start at one part of the river and then our bus would pick us up a mile or two downstream. I figured it couldn't drive all the way down to the riverbank, so getting to the bus without my leg would be difficult. I remember telling my parents that I didn't want to have to miss the trip.

"Miss the trip? Why would you have to do that?" my dad asked.

"Well, how else am I gunna do it?" I asked dramatically.

"Just keep it on."

"Da-ad, you know I can't do that. It'll ruin my leg. You totally don't understand my friends. They'll get hot and want to tip over the canoe just for the fun of it."

"Oh, I *totally* wouldn't understand, huh?" he said in a playfully mocking tone. "I mean, I was never a kid, so I wouldn't get it. But no, before you get your panties in a bunch, I was talking about using one of your old legs. I'll waterproof it for you," he said.

"Hmm, that might actually work. Do you even know how to do that?"

"You're questioning your old man?" he teased. "Of course, I can."

So, the next day he went to the hardware store and bought a bunch of waterproofing materials. He grabbed one of my old legs that I recently grew out of from my closet and took it into the garage. The garage was my dad's makeshift work area. It housed all his tools and had a bench for him to do whatever miscellaneous task he decided to tackle at the time. He decided to fill in the hole on the bottom of my foot with putty to ensure that no water could get in. The hole was about the size of a nickel and contained the screw that connected my foot to the socket. Then, he spritzed the entire outer socket with waterproofing spray. My dad saved the hardest task for last: creating a makeshift plastic bag shield to put over my knee so that water couldn't go down into the hollow socket.

Once again, my dad had come to my rescue. When I put it on to try it out, it was a little snug, but I knew it could get me through the short amount of time that I needed to wear it. Thankfully, when it came time to go on the trip, my friends didn't try to pull any stunts and tip the canoe. Therefore, we never got to test my dad's waterproofing skills. Regardless of the fact that it may or may not have been effective, I was much more appreciative of my dad just spending the time to do it for me. Just like he vowed from the beginning, he did anything it took to give me the same opportunities as all the other kids.

- - -

That same summer, the engineers had fabricated the foot that I helped design. They were calling it a Flex Foot. It was made of carbon and had an active heel that would flex upon impact. The carbon itself was more responsive and would provide a spring when I pushed off the toe. Some runners choose to wear the foot as is and not put a rubber foot shell or shoe over top of it in order to get the best motion possible, but I decided otherwise because it would be too slippery and wouldn't work on all the surfaces that I needed it to. Putting the foot shell over top of the Flex Foot dampened the responsiveness quite a bit, but I could still walk heel to toe better than I ever had before. I was excited to put the foot to the test to see how it could help me in sports.

The first chance to test out my foot was in volleyball. I went to a lot of open gyms and conditioning sessions at the Vandalia Butler High School Student Activity Center (SAC) in hopes of making the team. Although I had been involved in a lot of organized sports before, I had never been required to work as hard as I did at those conditioning sessions. The coaches instructed us to do box jumps, sprints (which we called suicides), and, worst of all, run a mile. Even though all the exercises were difficult, my leg didn't really hold me back. Sure, I was sore, but so was everyone else. Our muscles hadn't really been asked to perform those exact tasks before. But, running was a different story; it was always my nemesis.

It probably wouldn't have been as big of a deal if they didn't expect all the players to run a mile in under 7:30. We were told that we wouldn't make the team if we didn't run it in under that time. I remember thinking that it was so stupid to run a mile in volleyball. That's why I *chose* volleyball! You don't have to run long distances! Nonetheless, I knew griping about it wouldn't help anything. I still had to beat the time.

All the players would practice the mile once a week out at the track. The coaches would sit on stools at the finish line with stop watches and tell us our time. My friends would always be way ahead of me. I gave it all I had, but I was nowhere near my goal. In fact, at the beginning of the summer, I was almost a whole minute over.

Knowing that I wasn't going to accomplish the feat without working even harder, I asked my friend Jackie to run with me two additional times a week. Jackie lived in my neighborhood and was a much better runner (and volleyball player) than me. After telling my family what I wanted to do to practice, my mom got in her car and drove around our neighborhood in order to map out our running path by looking at her odometer. We found a route that was exactly a mile. Whenever Jackie and I would run together, I struggled to keep up with her and knew that she was trying to be nice by not leaving me behind. I timed myself during each run. I had shaved off a lot of time, but I still wasn't where I needed to be.

When tryouts came, I was apprehensive, knowing full well that I wouldn't be able to meet the coaches' expectations. We had to run around the track four times to equal a mile. I started out at a mild pace so that I wouldn't burn all my energy at the beginning. The first two laps were fairly easy, but the end was the challenging part. I hadn't thought about the exact reason that running was harder for me than everyone else, but now that I analyze it further, I assume a lot of energy was lost in the transfer since my foot didn't have any spring or response. Each time I took a step, some of the motion was dampened because I was unable to do the heel-toe movement.

Because of this, my face always turned beet red, and I tired out faster than the rest. When I finally reached the finish line, the head coach, Cheryl Stidham, shouted that I had made it in 7:46. I hadn't met the requirement. Shocking. Thinking that my fate was sealed, I dolefully headed back into the gym, totally defeated. I waited for my name to get called to go into one of the conference rooms in the SAC to be told that I didn't make the team. I sat on the gym floor growing more and more angry. Only, I wasn't angry at myself. I was furious that I had tried so hard to be told that I didn't make it based off a stupid mile time that had nothing to do with how well I could play volleyball. I had been pulled up to the eighth-grade team as a seventh grader. I had talent. Only a few girls hadn't made the mile time. But, those were girls who were not very athletic and had never played volleyball before. I had. My parents had told me time and time again that life wasn't fair, but I couldn't help wanting to be petty and scream, "But it's not fair!" at the coaches.

I had spent my entire life wanting to be like everyone else. Being treated the same was all I desired. But, this was the first time that I sought an exception for being an amputee. I wanted my coaches to give me a break, knowing that it was harder for me than everyone else. It was a double standard, I know. I wanted the best of both worlds: to be treated like everyone else, but also to be given exceptions when things got tough. I just wanted someone to verbally acknowledge the fact that my life was difficult and give me sympathy. I might have thought I wanted that at the time, but in hindsight, I am so glad that they didn't. It taught me much more that they held me to the same expectations as everyone else.

Suddenly, another player came back into the gym and said, "Kendra, they asked for you next."

I slowly walked back to the conference rooms and sat down in the chair that faced the two coaches. I was completely intimidated, not only due to the situation, but also of Coach Stidham. She was a force to be reckoned with; many of the freshman didn't like her (or maybe just weren't used to her) because she was fiery and didn't put up with anything. Don't get me wrong, she knew her volleyball, but she was our first experience with high school athletics, and she most definitely set the precedent. I wrung my hands and didn't make eye contact with them until coach Stidham asked, "How do you think your tryout went, Kendra?"

"Well, I didn't make the mile time." It was all I could think about. It wasn't like me to harp on my faults, but I knew this was a different caliber of play, and that I had failed to meet their expectations. It didn't matter that I was proud of my progress or that I had come to almost every single conditioning and open gym or that I knew I was better than about half of the other freshman. I figured all that mattered to them were the stats.

"Kendra, that's only one part of the tryout. We take everything into consideration. How do you think everything went as a whole?"

I was shocked. I thought it was a no brainer. I was just hoping that they would let me down easy, but I hadn't thought that they might overlook the mile. "Oh, um, I think I got a lot better this summer and my passing and serving is looking pretty good, but I would like to hit a little better. The ball keeps hitting the tape or it sails out past the end line a lot."

"Well, we've actually seen a lot of that too. You're the strongest server on the team. You definitely have that going for you, and you're not scared to dive for a ball."

"Wait, sorry, but did you say, 'on the team?'"

They looked at each other and laughed. "Yes, you made the freshman team."

"Really? But the mile..."

"Yeah, you didn't make it, but we appreciate the work that you put in to shave that much time off. If you're willing to work that hard for something, you're someone we want on our team."

I was elated! My hard work had paid off. In fact, as the season progressed, I won a starting spot on the team and played all the way around (both in the front row and back). My serving continued to be my strong suit. I would get on streaks where the other team really struggled to defend it in serve receive. Some games I scored ten or more points in a row because they had such trouble.

Although volleyball was going well, adjusting to high school was a different story. Thankfully, my sister was a senior, so she showed me the ropes. She helped me find all my classes and even let me share her locker for a couple transitions between classes since my locker was so far away.

At my high school, two different middle schools (Smith and Morton) merge together. I already had friends from Smith, but the rivalry between the two middle schools held strong, and I didn't really branch out and make any friends from Morton. Jackie was the only friend that I added to my friend group from a local private Catholic grade school because she and I had become close through volleyball.

Having friends helped a lot, but I still remember feeling very self-conscious. Initially, it was only due to a problem with my foot. The carbon Flex Foot had started to squeak for whatever reason. Every time I walked, it released this shrill, obnoxious noise. During class change, it wasn't that big of a deal because of the cacophony of a thousand or so teenage voices emanating from all directions, but if I needed to leave class to go to the bathroom or somewhere else, I was mortified. I tried whatever I could to not be in the echoing hallways alone without all the noise to mask the squeak. If, in an emergency situation, I took the chance and went, I *always* seemed to pass people, and they *always* seemed to be upperclassman. It wasn't just a fabrication of my mind. They stared at me. How could they not? It was loud! I wanted to offer up an excuse or reason when I passed people to try to let them know what was happening, but it was way too long of a story, and I didn't even know where to start. So, I just hung my head in embarrassment and walked as quickly as I could to get it over with. You can imagine how my fast pace amplified the sound even more.

My parents told me that the foot might just need to break in a bit. They thought the newness of it might be causing it to squeak. But, after a couple weeks of dealing with it, I couldn't bear it any longer. I sat down on my couch and started bawling my eyes out. My mom consoled me and did what any good mother does—told me it was going to be ok. My dad, like most men, just wanted to find a solution to the problem. No one wanted to make the trek down to Kentucky again, so he went all MacGyver on it and took it apart. When he did, my dad saw that the toe area was causing the problem. The carbon was split into two sections at that location and the pieces were rubbing together for some reason. He jammed some soft fabric pieces in between so that it couldn't create any friction. With the squeak now gone, we thought that he'd fixed the issue, but a volleyball game or two later, we discovered otherwise.

About halfway through the game, while playing outside hitter, my setter set me a perfect ball. I spiked it, but when landing back on the floor, I could tell that something wasn't right. I felt a vibration of sorts and heard something snap as I fell to the hard, gym floor. I tried to get back up, but when I did, I could immediately tell that my foot couldn't support all of my weight. The athletic trainer came out onto the floor and had me put my arm around his neck so that he could help support me as I hobbled to the bench. Because I wasn't actually hurt, and it was way more to do with my prosthesis, the trainer motioned to my mom, who was thankfully in the stands for every home match. I took my foot shell off and saw that the carbon flex foot had completely snapped in half. So much for it being more durable and robust.

Therefore, another trip to The Shriners Medical Center ensued. I was more frustrated by the timing of it than anything. Since it happened during the season, I had to miss school to drive all the way to Lexington. But, Vandalia Butler, like most area schools, had a rule that players had to be at school at least half the day in order to play in their game or match. So, our long, drawn out family vacation style trips stopped happening. Instead, they were replaced with even earlier than normal wake up calls, quick driving, and lunch on the go while I took a nap so I could stay awake in my classes for the second half of the day.

The season went on without any other problems. In fact, my foot never broke like that again. It must have just been a fluke or maybe I landed in exactly a way that put too much stress on the weakest part. But, thankfully, it held up much better after that incident.

By the end of the season, I could see that the other girls were starting to get just as good if not better at hitting than me. A lot of them were my same height, but because they could jump higher than me, they hit the ball better. My coach would always tell me to jump off of both legs, but using my right leg to jump only hindered me. I tried to use every other part of my body to help me get some spring and height, but I couldn't compensate enough. Knowing that I was pretty much done growing and that I probably wouldn't be able to jump much higher, I started to doubt how well I would do at the Junior Varsity level the next year when the competition was even harder.

At the conclusion of the season, each player had a one on one meeting with Coach Stidham to discuss the season and to talk about plans for the summer.

"So, Kendra, are you happy with how the season went?"

"Yeah, for the most part. I liked how much playing time I got, and I had a lot of fun. I still wish I could hit better.

"Yeah, your team had a lot of success and a great record. Have you thought about trying out for club?"

"Oh, uh, not really. I play softball in the summer, and my parents can't really afford club. We've heard it's really expensive."

"Well, you know that while you are taking the summer off, the other players will be playing club and improving their skills. If you don't play, you will likely not be a starter on JV. You might have trouble even making the team to be honest."

Talk about taking the wind out of my sails! I was instantly deflated. Knowing that the other players were already catching up to me coupled by the fact the coaches seemed to already have their minds made up about the next season, I decided right then and there that I was done with volleyball.

That was the first time that I ever gave up on anything. I let Stidham's words tear me down instead of give me the drive to prove her wrong. Do I regret not trying out the next year? Absolutely! However, some good did come from the situation. I was bound and determined from that point forward to prove to any naysayers that I could do anything (especially if they told me I couldn't).

Chapter 9

Amputee Realities that are Often Overlooked

After a growth spurt around my sophomore year in high school, it was time to be fitted for yet another prosthesis. Although, this time was a bit different. Wayne told me about a new procedure that involved answering a set of questions on my ability level and mobility. He said it was a sort of ranking system to determine what type of prosthesis was the most practical for each patient. After assessing my current level, he would be able to justify obtaining a different, more versatile leg for me.

The Shriners Medical Center is still using this same ranking system today. Patients can be classified anywhere between a K1-K4. Eric Miller stated that, "A K1 patient would have limited mobility and might struggle doing typical daily tasks such as sitting down in a chair and getting back up without holding onto something. A K2 would have the potential for ambulation with the ability to walk well on flat surfaces, go up small inclines, or go up and down stairs. A K3 would walk with variable cadence and speed, would adjust to different surfaces, and have a relatively smooth gait. Lastly, a K4 would be able to endure significant impact (such as running and jumping) and could do athletic movements with ease."

Wayne asked me roughly twenty questions. After totaling up the number of points I received, he determined that I was a K4. My score warranted a more durable, high tech prosthesis than some other patients needed.

From the assessment, it was decided that I qualified for a locking liner suspension instead of semi-suction in hopes of my prosthesis staying on better while doing physical activities. I was told that this new liner would be made of silicone on the inside and a fabric-like material on the outside. It would have to be turned inside out and then placed on the bulbous end of my stump before being tightly rolled up to slightly above my knee. The outside of the liner would have a screw attached to the bottom. That screw would fit inside of a locking mechanism on the inside of the socket. The prosthesis couldn't come off unless a button on the outside of my leg was pushed to release the screw (which is also called a pin).

Needless to say, I couldn't wait to get the call from Wayne telling me that it was ready to be picked up. I hoped, with much anticipation, that it would give me more comfort and help me perform better in sports.

Upon retrieval, I noticed an instant change: the weight. The locking pin suspension was a lot lighter. It felt amazing to not have to carry around that much weight anymore. I hadn't ever noticed how heavy it was until I put on the new socket. I guess I never knew what I was missing. Wayne had even surprised me with a last-minute change. He had switched the outer foot shell to one with a split toe, which meant there was a gap between my big toe and second toe. Instantly, I knew why the gap was there.

"I can wear flip flops now!" I shouted enthusiastically. "Mom, we *have* to go shopping."

She smiled widely, showing off her crow's feet that she was always complaining about. It seemed as if she was vicariously experiencing my joy right with me.

Non-amputees probably don't think twice about putting on a pair of flip flops. Imagine having to traipse through a sandy beach with gym shoes that fill up with copious amounts of sand or spending time putting shoes on and tying them in the summer when other people can simply slip on some sandals. That was my reality. Now that I was able to wear flip flops, it was a luxury that I vowed to never take for granted.

Not only did we stop at an outlet mall on the way home to get several new pairs, but I begged my parents to have my friends over for a sleepover that night so that I could show them my new leg. My friends took turns trying to pull my leg off, which, in hindsight, probably wasn't one of my smartest moves. They were amazed at how hard they could tug without it coming off, and conversely, how easily it released when they pushed the button.

After the acclimation period was over and I started to feel comfortable in the new socket, I started to notice that I had subconsciously held back when running and had developed certain habits like flexing my stump in order to keep my prosthesis on. With the new socket, I ran without any hesitation like never before. I wasn't concerned about it coming off; therefore, I didn't have to nurse it in any fashion. My speed and agility improved, as did my confidence.

- - -

Even though I was now able to wear flip flops, buying shoes was a more challenging endeavor than most people experience. I still couldn't wear high heels. My foot couldn't adjust to withstand the additional heel height, so if I tried to wear them, they just sent my knee forward and messed up my alignment. It wasn't comfortable to walk, and I looked like a fool doing it.

When the homecoming dance came around and it was time to go dress shopping, I wasn't as excited as all my other friends. The dress part wasn't the problem; it was the shoes. My mom took me to one of the department stores at the Dayton Mall and was ever so patient.

"How about these?" she asked as she held up a pair of black flats next to my new black and white, knee-length dress.

"Mom, I know you're trying, but none of these are going to look good. Dresses look stupid with flats."

"Well, heels aren't an option for you, so we're just going to have to find the cutest flats in this store."

I didn't give her enough credit. She had so much empathy and never got frustrated with me. We would spend an hour in one store looking at shoes, none of which were for her. She rarely shopped for herself. That was mostly because she was frugal, but shopping just wasn't her thing.

"Kendra, come look at these," she said in her normal, even tone. However, because I knew her so well, I picked up on the subtle excitement even from a few rows away. I quickly walked in the direction of her voice. When I saw what she was holding, I rushed up to them to inspect them further. They had about a half inch heel, but since it was so minute, I thought that they might actually work.

I took my sock off and eagerly put the black, strappy heel onto my artificial foot. I knew it would fit since it was a size 10, but that wasn't the issue. Would I be able to walk naturally in them? I practiced walking through the aisles. The heel height didn't bother me, but I wondered how I looked.

"Wow, you actually walk pretty well in them," my mom said. "I mean, when you're just standing there, I can tell that your knee sticks out a bit, but when you walk, I can't even tell. It looks pretty natural."

"Really? Oh my gosh. Mom, I'm actually wearing heels!"

She chuckled and started to package everything back into the box while I took them off. She started to head to the counter.

"Wait. Don't I have to pay for those?"

"Not this time. This is a special day." My mom wasn't only the most economically savvy person that I had ever met, but she also tried to impress upon us the value of a dollar. When I had saved up the $50 that was necessary to start a savings account, she drove me clear across town to the bank. 10% had to go to church. At least 10% had to be saved, and the other 80% went to paying for extras. Because, being only a sophomore, I wasn't exactly rolling in the dough, my parents paid for things that I needed, while I was expected to pick up the items I wanted. The exception that she made that day was duly noted. Who knew that finding a pair of heels could be so impactful? But, as an amputee, it meant the world to me.

-   -   -

I know fashion isn't the most important thing when discussing the complications that many amputees have. But to a teenage girl, it was pretty high on my priority list. However, what made me even more angry is how my athletic ability was limited no matter how hard I tried to mentally overcome it.

I made the Junior Varsity softball team my sophomore year. The previous year, I started on the Freshman team only to be moved up to JV halfway through the season. The JV coach saw how well my friend Andrea and I were doing and decided that we had the talent to succeed at a higher level of competition. During preseason conditioning in the gym, my coach, Bob Dadey, was hitting at us so that we could practice fielding the ball. The ball would quickly skid across the wood floor at a much faster pace than it would have on a dirt field. I knew if I could field the balls that he fired at us indoors, I would be able to successfully do it outside.

I stood my ground on our makeshift field and tried not to flinch as the ball whizzed towards me at superspeed. The whole team did this endlessly, practicing so often to develop muscle memory. I would dive on the floor in hopes of getting a ball that was just out of reach, my skin screeching against the hardwood. After reconnecting with my old coach, I was pleased to hear that he remembered (despite 17 years passing) how hard I tried: "You always gave it everything you had in practice. You had a never-quit attitude and never said you couldn't do something. Your work ethic and positive attitude seemed to rub off on the other players." As a consequence of playing with that much heart, my body was riddled with aches and pains.

When practice was over one day, my teammates and I sat down in a circle to stretch and cool down. After about two minutes, I just couldn't take it anymore. My leg was swollen, sweaty, and sore, so I decided to push the button on the interior side of my prosthesis and take it off to give it a rest.

Bob remembers that day very well: "I knew you had a prosthetic leg from the knee down and I had seen the prosthesis when you would be at practice. What I had never seen was the prosthesis *off* of your leg. I remember the first time I had seen it as if it were yesterday. We had just concluded practice in the central gym and like most practices, I ended it with running. When everyone was finished running, I met with the team and most of the players were sitting on the gym floor. As I began to talk, I looked down and saw that you had removed your prosthetic leg. I would not say I was shocked by it, but it was definitely out of the norm for me and it took me a moment to process what I was looking at. You just sat there smiling because you knew by the look on my face that I was not accustomed to seeing this! And of course, you had the other girls laughing!"

Taking my leg off in this fashion did not warrant the same reaction from me as the pool or other situations where I felt self-conscious. This was different; it was a group of girls, many of whom I had played softball with for years. I was comfortable with them, so when it hurt, I didn't think twice about removing it.

It was that season that I got another little taste of how my leg was starting to hold me back and the competition grew more intense. I had always rotated my time between second base and catcher, but after training so hard during the off-season, I still lost out on not only the starting catcher role, but I hardly ever got to even play as the backup. The girl that beat me out at the position was Andrea Franceschelli. I knew even then that my coach made the right decision. I hated to admit it, but she was better than me. We both had pretty good arms for throwing it down to second, but she could trap balls better than me because of her side to side agility while in the squatting position.

Because the back of my prosthesis goes up right to where the knee bends, my movement was restricted. It served a lot of good purposes like supporting my weaker and smaller than normal knee, but when it came to agility, I couldn't bend it as well as I needed to. When our pitcher threw a wild pitch, it was Andrea that could get to the ball faster. In previous seasons, this wasn't a problem because the pitcher didn't have as much speed, but now that she was throwing faster, I couldn't get to the ball as well.

Mentally, that was a difficult thing to handle. I knew what I needed to do, but that didn't seem to matter. Trying harder than most girls on the team only got me so far. Of course, no one would ever tell me that my leg was the thing holding me back for fear of being offensive, but they didn't have to. I knew. That was the worst part about it. No matter what I did or how hard I tried, I just couldn't make up for my deficit. I was way too headstrong to be ok with that, but I did have to learn to accept it on some levels.

- - -

Driving was another thing that was more difficult because of my prosthesis. That January, when I turned fifteen and a half, I got my temps. Because my mom was a nervous person by nature, my dad mostly took on the burden of teaching me to drive. He took me to the sports complex by my house so that I could ease into the process by starting out in a parking lot rather than a road. Driving is a difficult skill for most teenagers to master, but add an artificial right leg to the equation and things got complicated quickly.

My dad pulled into a parking spot and switched places with me, putting me behind the wheel.

"Ok, now, the car is off, so it's not goin' anywhere," my dad explained. "What I want you to do is move your foot back and forth from the break to the gas a few times so you can just get a feel for it."

I did as he instructed.

"Good. Now, can you feel the pedal with your foot?"

"Nope. Not at all. I can tell when I'm on it though. I don't know how to explain it, but I know when I touch it. Maybe it's the vibration or something."

"Hmm…well, why don't we just take the car to my shop. I can switch the pedals and you can drive with your left foot instead."

"No. I want to try it like this first. I think I can do it."

"But, Kendra, we need to make sure we're being safe here. For you and the other drivers."

"I know, but I really think I can do this. No one is in this parking lot, Dad. This is the perfect spot for me to try it."

This was just another example of how I avoided being different than other people at all costs. Switching the pedals meant giving in, relinquishing control.

"Ok, fine. We'll try it a couple times, but if it doesn't work out, I'm switching them," my dad said.

"Deal."

"Alright, I'm going to back it out of this spot, and you'll take over. I want you to just let your foot off the break this time. Don't touch the gas at all. It's gunna start to roll, and that's what we want.

99

Near the end of this section, put your foot back on the break and put the car into park."

"Got it," I said nervously as my knuckles turned white from gripping the steering wheel so tightly.

Everything went smoothly. I did just as he said, and when he felt confident that I knew what I was doing, he let me start pushing the gas, making turns, and even push the speed up to 15 mph.

I practiced for the required six months until I could get my license. A few days before I was scheduled to take my driver's test, Jackie was dropping me off at my house after a summer shopping excursion. She was almost a year older than me even though we were in the same grade, putting us both almost ready to start our junior year. As soon as we made the right turn onto Ronald Street, I could see a strange car in my driveway. It was an old, rundown, royal blue Chevrolet Beretta with two doors. Right away, I knew that jalopy was mine. My dad had been talking about buying me a car, and we had worked out a deal: he would buy the car and do the normal maintenance on it, but I had to pay for the gas, insurance, and repairs.

When comparing it to Jackie's car, it looked like a hooptie. She had a new forest green Sunfire. On top of that, it was a convertible. But, I didn't care. Although I appreciated how cool her car was, I really wasn't jealous. It was a free car. How could I complain about that? I was well aware that my parents couldn't afford anything nicer, and I always thought it was stupid for high schoolers to own brand new cars that they would probably wreck within a year.

I ran into the house, dropped my bookbag in the middle of the foyer, and shouted, "Mom? Where are you?"

"In here," she shouted from the kitchen.

"It's mine, isn't it?"

"What's yours?" she asked coyly.

"Mo-om," I said, breaking the monosyllabic word into two. "Don't play dumb. The car in the driveway… is it mine?"

"Oh, you put two and two together, huh?" she said, laughing. "Yes. But with it comes responsibility," she went on to lecture.

"I know. I know. But, it's really mine? Thank you thank you thank you," I said in rapid succession.

"You're welcome, but your father and I have already talked, and we don't want you driving it until you get used to it. Every car is different, and since you can't feel the pedals, you're going to have to relearn where they are in your car.

"Ok, that's fine," I said, willing to do whatever it took for it to become mine.

I obviously don't know how driving feels to "normal" people, but after I gained more experience, it came to my attention that finding the pedals wasn't the only thing that was harder about driving for me. My foot doesn't swivel when going back and forth from the break and the gas the way most people's do. Because of this, I have to lift my whole leg up and over to transition between the two. My foot doesn't move forward and back either, so I can't push on the pedals the same way. I have to use my entire leg to push instead of moving my ankle. This makes long drives very tiring. My 1990 Chevy Beretta didn't have cruise control, so that made it even tougher. Traffic jams are the worst! During stop and go traffic, I often place my hand under my right hamstring to help lift my leg if my muscles get fatigued. Or, during a stop, I quickly move my left foot over to the break to give my right leg a rest.

Additionally, it is hard to determine how fast I am going. I can't really tell how hard I push the gas, so I am constantly looking down at my speedometer to gauge my speed. All of this seems challenging, but I really have adjusted well. I have come to determine that people can do a lot more than they think they can. Our bodies have a way of adapting. Maybe it's better that I don't know what it's like for other people to drive. I'm not privy to how easy it is for them, so adjusting to driving the way that I do is just second nature.

Driving only became an issue one time in high school. A few months after I had my license, I was sitting in the Vandalia Butler school parking lot after school released a little after two in the afternoon. The parking lot was a madhouse with approximately 500 cars all trying to get out of two exits. I got into the line and tried to patiently wait my turn. But, it was raining that day, and I was wearing the new pair of heels that I got with my mom. To everyone else, that wouldn't be a big deal, but for me, the mixture of rain and slippery soles made for quite the debacle.

My foot slipped off the break. I couldn't find the pedal again right away because I wasn't used to my foot being on the floorboard instead of a pedal. I had to take my eyes off the car in front of me while I looked under my dash to locate the break. In doing so, I hit the car in front of me. After putting my car in park, I stepped out and walked up to the driver's side window of the car I hit. When the window started rolling down, I discovered that it was a girl that I played softball with, Chelsey. Although I knew Chelsey from being on the team, she and I weren't exactly friends.

"Oh my gosh. I am so sorry. Are you ok?" I asked. I was mortified. All the nearby drivers who had witnessed the wreck were staring at me, intrigued by the action.

"Yeah, I'm fine. What were you doing?" I could tell she was flustered, probably even a bit pissed off if I would have had to guess. I looked at the back of her car, and there was only slight damage. Some of the paint had chipped off, but there weren't any dents. It really could have been much worse. Thankfully, I was only going at parking lot speed.

I told her what had happened and then asked, "So, what do we do now? I give you my insurance info, right?"

"Yeah, I guess."

I scribbled the information on a piece of paper and gave it to her. We also exchanged phone numbers. I rushed back into my car, very shaken up. All sorts of things were running through my head: it was my fault, my parents were going to be furious, and how was I going to pay for the repairs? I drove home restraining the tears that wanted so desperately to come out.

When I pulled into my driveway, my tears won, no longer able to be stifled. When I opened the door in the garage that lead into the house, my mom heard my sobs.

"Kendra? What's wrong?" I was crying so hard that I couldn't formulate words. My mom was panicked. "Are you hurt?

What happened?" Her questions came out like bullets from a machine gun.

Finally, I had settled down enough to say, "I wrecked my car."

"Oh boy." Her tone immediately changed to calm and sympathetic. "Well, you don't seem hurt. Is the other person ok?"

"Yeah. It happened in the school parking lot. My car is totally fine, but hers has some paint missing. I'm so sorry. My shoe was wet from the rain and it slipped off the pedal. I just couldn't find it in time."

She went out to look at the damage and saw that my car was completely unscathed. "Well, you got lucky. No one was hurt. That's what matters."

"Yeah, but what about her car? Won't this make my insurance go up? How am I going to pay for this?" Tears started to come again, but this time they fell silently down my cheeks.

"Whoa, hold on. Let me call your dad. I think he should know about all of this, and we'll come up with a game plan, ok?" said my mom.

"You're not mad?"

"Well, I'm not exactly thrilled, but part of me knows that you couldn't really help it."

It was a long, agonizing wait for my dad to get home from work. My dad was normally the one that was more understanding of my sister and I's infractions. He hadn't exactly been an angel when he was a kid, so I think he was more accepting of our faults than my mom was. But, I knew my dad had a different side to him that didn't come out very often. You see, when my dad did get angry, he would go to extremes and ground us for a month. My mom would plead for him to reduce the sentence because she said it was punishing her too, having to be in the house with us all the time with no privileges. My mom took care of the day-to-day discipline, so her punishments were less severe. So, in short, we knew not to piss Dad off.

I had no idea how he would react to this one. The fact that my mom wasn't that upset led me to believe that there was a glimmer of hope. So, when he walked through the door, I stayed on the family room couch and was completely silent. I thought it was better to have him start the conversation.

The second that he came over to me, sat beside me, and kissed me on the forehead, I knew all was well. "Hey Pooh, I heard ya had a bit of a rough day, huh?"

"Yeah, you could say that."

"Well, your mom and I spoke, and here's what we're going to do. I already called Chelsey's dad. Since it was on private property, he has agreed to bring his car into my shop and have us repair her car. We aren't going to get the insurance companies involved. That'll help keep the cost down."

"How much do you think it will cost to fix her car?"

"From what her dad said, it's not too bad, so not much. Your mom and I agreed that we'll pay for half of the repair because your leg was mostly at fault. You have to pay the other half though."

"Thanks, Dad," I said, wrapping my arms around his neck.

After hearing our conversation come to a close, my mom made her way into the room. "Tim, you forgot to mention our new rule."

"Oh yeah. We don't want you wearing dress shoes when you drive anymore. If you ever need to wear them somewhere, you'll have to pack them."

"Maybe just throw a pair of your old gym shoes into the back of your car so that you're prepared," my mom suggested. "But, I think you learned a valuable lesson today about wearing appropriate driving shoes. None of us thought about it before this, but now that we know it's an issue, we need to make sure it doesn't happen again."

"Yeah, that's probably a good idea. I can definitely do that."

Although I kept my portion of the agreement all throughout high school, I have to admit that once I got to college, I didn't pack a change of shoes anymore. Maybe I got cocky or maybe I gained enough experience that I didn't really need to. Either way, I haven't caused an accident since.

Chapter 10

Leaning on the Support of Others

After quitting volleyball, I decided to dabble in tennis for a couple years. I had always grown up playing with my parents at Helke Park. The tennis courts were adjacent to my elementary school and were within walking distance of my house. When I was really young and too uncoordinated to play, I would tag along and act as my parents' ball girl as they played against each other for exercise.

I never had any training other than that, so when my friends asked me to come out for the team, I was skeptical to say the least. I decided to go to the summer conditionings so that I could scope out my competition. I wanted to hang out with my friends, but I didn't want to play JV as a junior, or even worse, get cut from the team. That wouldn't do much to help my ego. But, what I soon discovered was that it was nothing like volleyball. It wasn't so cutthroat; the whole environment was much more relaxed. Many of the girls were new to the sport, and because I was fairly athletic, I was able to pick up on the basics pretty quickly.

I loved everything about tennis: the uniforms (a cute tank top and skirt), being outdoors in the warm weather, the shorter matches, and the fact that it was more of an individual sport. I liked not having to rely on anyone else. If I had a bad game, it was no one's fault other than mine. I was always intrinsically motivated, so I really started to thrive.

I surprisingly made Varsity my junior year and played third singles. That year I developed a mean topspin forehand, and I was very consistent with my backhand, a feat that many people struggle with. I worked the angles well and had a fast serve that many people had trouble returning. Don't get me wrong, I still had a lot to learn, but I improved quickly.

However, my leg came into play once again. My new locking liner didn't let my skin breathe very well. The sweat would pool up in the bottom of the liner, and it would slowly start to slide down my stump. Through this process, my leg would sit lower than normal in the socket. Places that weren't used to the friction or hadn't developed calluses were then being rubbed against, which caused me a lot of pain. If it got too wet, then my whole prosthesis could come right off, but I never let it get to that point. Instead, I would take it off every single time my opponent and I switched sides between sets. I carried a towel in my bag and would dry it off quickly before putting it back on. When I took the liner off, about a half an inch of sweat would pour out of it, creating a puddle on the green, acrylic-covered asphalt.

I never really noticed or cared what my opponent thought about my leg or the fact that I had just put on quite a unique show. In the two years that I played tennis, not one single player ever said one word to me about it. I know they saw it; it was too out of the ordinary to miss. I just think they either were too shocked for words or they had no idea what to say. I was way more concerned with winning the match anyway. I didn't care about niceties or being embarrassed; I was never embarrassed about being an amputee around girls. No one seemed to pity me or go easy on me, which I respected. I didn't want any excuses. My competitive nature wouldn't allow for that.

Although I was decent at singles, the next season my coach, John Kuhns, suggested that I try doubles. I didn't have to move as much, which helped the sweatiness factor. My friend, Jessi Hope, who played second singles the year before, and I decided to partner up and try our hand at first doubles on the Varsity team. She was better than me since she took private lessons and was more technically trained. But, what I lacked in skill, I made up for with heart and determination. Jessi didn't really have the competitive gene that I seemed to possess, but together, we started to win a lot of matches. We got honorable mention and made it fairly far in the tournament. My memory fails me now, but I know we got past sectionals.

It was during one of those tournament matches when the coach from the other team came up and started talking to Coach Kuhns right behind the fence of court number four where we were playing. I didn't think much of it at the time, figuring they were just socializing to pass the time. But after the match, my coach came up to me and put his arm around my sweaty shoulders.

"You see that coach over there?" Coach Kuhns asked.

"Yeah."

"He is very impressed with you. He can't believe you're an amputee. He saw you lay out for a ball a few times this match and just loved how much you play with your heart."

"Aww. That's nice," I said, my cheeks growing flush from the compliment.

"Kendra, you truly are special. I told him I didn't have anyone on the team like you. If everyone worked as hard as you, we would win the GMC. But, then he asked if you were going anywhere to play in college—"

"Ha. Nope, not good enough for that," I said, shutting the idea down immediately.

"Well, I don't know. No one offered you a scholarship, but so what? Maybe you could walk on somewhere."

It was nice to hear that someone recognized my hard work and truly believed in my ability. He gave his affirmation in such a way that I actually started to believe it myself. Coach Kuhns' support boosted my confidence and made me play even harder, hoping not to let him down.

After briefly considering playing in college, I realized that it was a long shot, and I didn't really want to devote the necessary time to a college sport anyway. However, I loved the game, and continued to play leisurely through adulthood... never without a sweat towel nearby of course.

- - -

My mom loved to travel, and that rubbed off on the rest of my family. It was her goal to visit all 50 states before she died. Unfortunately, she didn't quite meet her goal, but she was darn close. I think we all came to an agreement during her memorial service that it was around 34, give or take one or two. Ever since my parents had kids, they vowed to take a summer vacation each year. Now, like I said before, we weren't rich by any means. My mom jokingly told us at dinner one night that her highest annual salary was $24,000. It wasn't a lot, but with their combined income, they saved enough to go on a beach vacation every other year. The years in between we would normally go on a day trip to somewhere close by or maybe stay a night or two, depending on how much extra money we had that year.

The summer of my Junior year happened to be beach year. We had gone to Panama City Beach, Florida once before, but we loved it so much that we wanted to go back. Even though my sister was in college, she went with us. During our week's stay, we would go to the beach in the mornings, go back to our hotel room for lunch and a quick break from the sun, and then go back out to the pool in the afternoon. We would come in around 3:00 so that everyone could shower and go out to dinner. We finished each night with some type of family activity like miniature golf. Those vacations really were the best of times and succeeded in bringing our already tight-knit family even closer.

But, what should have been a relaxing, stress-free trip quickly turned into the exact opposite (at least for a few hours anyway). Rachel and I loved laying out by the pool. We were old enough that my parents didn't really hover around all the time; they knew that we wanted our space. We had started talking to these two boys by the pool. Again, I loved attention from guys and searched for any occasion to hear that I was pretty to put my insecure thoughts at bay for even a little while. I even lied to one of them and said that I was two years older than I was. Both guys were around my sister's age, and I wanted nothing more than to seem cool or to fit in with them. I know that this makes me look desperate and pathetic, but it's the extent that I would go to seek male approval. Thankfully, I knew where to draw the line with this game and didn't push too far physically. My Christian upbringing really helped with that and gave me an excuse to not cross certain lines. I didn't need all of that anyways. Once I won the guy over and heard what I wanted to hear or got the attention I was seeking, I was off to hear it from someone else.

Over the next few days, we flirted with the two guys whenever we happened to cross paths, which was fairly often since they were staying at the same hotel. Another group of five girls our age came a couple days into our stay. We had already met the two boys and established our "territory" if you will. We could tell that the girls hated us because we had the boy's attention and they didn't. There really weren't any other guys our age, so they were out of luck, and not happy about it. They did everything they could to express their discontent: rolled their eyes, walked in front of us all too often, gathered in a circle and giggled and then looked in our direction while laughing. Basically, any normal petty things that teenage girls do to establish their dominance, they did.

Rachel and I didn't really think anything of it. It was typical behavior that we were accustomed to. We weren't all that invested in the guys anyway. They just kept us company during our short stay. They didn't even live in the same state, so we were just trying to have some innocent fun.

But, things got serious pretty quickly. My family was in our hotel room eating lunch. Afterwards, I stepped out onto the balcony that overlooked the pool to relax and read a book. I was completely engrossed, but when I heard a lot of loud noises below, my eyes diverted their attention away from my book long enough to satisfy my curiosity. There was the group of girls. They were standing in the pool, crowded around something that I couldn't quite make out. They were pointing up at me and then down at the object.

Standing up, I set my book on the outdoor table that was next to my patio chair. I got up close to the balcony railing and squinted to get a better look. There, floating on top of the water, was a fake, rubber hand. At first, I didn't get it, but I knew they had ill intentions. After a couple seconds, it dawned on me that they were mocking my prosthesis. I didn't utter a word or give them the satisfaction of getting a rise out of me. I simply opened the sliding glass door and called for my sister.

"Rache, come here a sec."

She was laying on one of the beds watching tv, almost asleep. I could tell she was instantly annoyed by my beckon. "What do you want? I'm comfy."

"Just come here please." She must have picked up that something was going on because she stood up and walked out onto the balcony. "Look what those girls put in the pool."

"You've got to be kidding me! Where the hell would they have gotten a fake hand?"

"Ha, beats me. But, I guess they didn't sell feet," I joked.

By this time, my mom had made her way out there too. We clued her in and I could instantly see her start to get fired up. As soon as they saw my mom come out onto the balcony, they snatched the hand out of the water and quickly got out of the pool.

"I'm going down there," said my mom.

"Whoa whoa whoa. No, you're not. Mom, please!" I begged. "That would be so embarrassing."

"Who cares. Those girls need to know what they did was wrong."

"Just let it go, Mom. It's fine. They're just stupid girls."

"Sorry, but I have to." I knew what she meant. She needed to teach them a lesson, but more importantly, she had to stand up for her daughter. I just let her go. Rachel and I stayed put right there on the balcony so we could have a good view of the show.

My mom finally made her way down to the pool and instantly confronted the group as they were toweling off. I have no idea what she said because we were out of earshot, but her animated body language allowed us to fill in the gaps. At that moment, I was both mortified and proud. My mom always took other people's sides and encouraged me to see things from other's viewpoints at all cost. It was aggravating and made me doubt where her allegiance lied. But on this occasion, she let her fiery side come out. I appreciated her standing up for me more because she never did. However, to her credit, that is the first time I really allowed her to step in and come to my aid.

When she came back up to the room, I just shook my head and asked, "What'd ya say?"

"I told them that they were rude and that they could spend their time doing something productive rather than exploit people's differences. I also demanded that they apologize to you, so let me know if they don't."

"Oh my gosh, Mom. I can't believe you just did that." My whole family started dying laughing.

My dad went over to her and put his arm around her shoulders. "You let that redheaded attitude come out, huh?" She didn't say anything in return, but her smile spoke volumes.

About an hour later, my family went down to the pool together. We pulled four chairs together, sat our stuff down, and started to relax. About ten minutes in, I caught a glimpse of the group of girls. They were walking straight toward me, but instead of their arrogant, sassy countenance, they looked like a guilty puppy right after he pees on the floor. One of the girls apologized on the group's behalf and the others echoed their "yeah, we're sorry's." I couldn't believe that they had actually followed through and heeded my mom's instructions. Maybe she had scared the bejesus out of them or maybe they had hearts enough to know they were wrong after all. They definitely didn't have to apologize. There wasn't really any way for my mom to make them, but they had done it. And for that, I'll give them some credit.

I thought that the immature, hurtful comments were a thing of the past when I exited middle school, but I guess some people never really grow out of it. And, I'm not too naive to think that I was their only victim. Anyone who stands out as being different has a huge target on his/her back. I just so happened to be one of them. That kind of intolerance, though, I will never understand. Those girls went out of their way to drive to a store and gather ammunition to load their gun of hatred. That day I learned the depth of people's enmity and malice. With that being said, I have thankfully come to realize there are way more good people in this world than bad.

- - -

As Junior year came to a close, I started thinking more about college. Not only was I going on college visits, but I was scoping out any type of financial aid I could get. After determining Education was going to be my major, I applied for a ton of scholarships. I knew that my family fell right into the category of making too much money to get any kind of governmental assistance and not making enough to pay for it outright. My parents had paid for half of Rachel's college tuition, so I figured they would do the same for me. But, I didn't have enough saved up to pay for the remainder of my portion. That's when my mom did what any normal person would do that is in search of answers. She went to the internet.

On one of her searches, she discovered an organization called the Bureau of Vocational Rehabilitation (BVR). Their website boasted "Opportunities for Ohioans with disabilities." Unsure of everything they had to offer and if I even qualified for their services, my mom set up a meeting with them to get more information.

During that initial meeting in downtown Dayton, the person we spoke to was very optimistic that I would not only qualify, but that they would be able to help reduce the financial burden of college substantially. After being asked a series of questions, I started feeling a little uneasy. Questions like, "Do you need help getting in and out of the shower? Do you require assistance to get to class? What special accommodations do you need for your dorm room?" were what caused me to have this reaction. I answered the questions honestly, but everything that I said, they seemed to spin into me requiring more aid. For example, they would say, "Well, what if your leg broke? Would you need assistance then?" I just felt like I would be dishonestly taking funds away from people who actually needed help. We picked up an application as we left, but I was pretty sure that I would not be accepting their help.

On the way home, I vividly remember expressing my guilt and hesitancy to my mom.

"Mom, I just can't take their money."

"Honey, I see where you're coming from, but I think sometimes you forget that the cards are stacked against you. You do have it very well. You are fortunate, but that's when you compare yourself to other people with physical limitations. What about people who don't have any?"

"Yeah, I guess. But why should me being an amputee get me money for school?"

"This organization is devoted to evening the playing field so that people like you can have an equal shot at getting good, quality jobs. These days, it's hard to do that without attending college. They're just helping you get to your end goal."

"Yeah, and I'm glad there are organizations out there like that, but I'm going to college either way, regardless of how much they help me. So, I don't really *need* their help."

"Kendra, life is a balancing act. It's time things went your way a bit and for you to get rewarded for all of your hard work and perseverance. Don't be too prideful. Let someone help you for once. It's good to be stubborn. It's helped you through so many things, but you have to know when to stop making it harder on yourself just for the sake of it. Does that make sense?"

I couldn't really argue with what she said. It was my first of many lessons in dispelling my pride. In fact, it's something that I still struggle with today. Whether I liked it or not, BVR changed my life. Not only did I get accepted, but they paid for most of my tuition, all my books, and half my room and board my first year. My parents didn't even have to pay their portion that they agreed to pay because, with my academic scholarship added in, we owed absolutely nothing. Because BVR's funds began to run out, I got less and less each year, but they always were able to provide me with some type of assistance.

I would not be as financially stable today if BVR hadn't helped me. Like most college students, I would have come out after four years burdened with debt that would take years to pay back. But, I graduated with zero debt. Zero! I still don't know if I deserved it or if it was right to take the money, but what I do know is that I am forever grateful for that organization.

Chapter 11

Early Adulthood: Embracing my Uniqueness

Just after turning 18, I entered my freshman year at The University of Toledo. I chose the school for many different reasons: the campus was beautiful, it was two hours away (close enough to my hometown to visit for the weekend but far enough away to give me the freedom that I wanted), and they gave me the most scholarship money. Rachel went there too, so I felt very comfortable, having visited her numerous times.

With much anticipation, I waited to move into college. I was both excited and nervous since I didn't know my roommate. She and I had emailed a few times after getting each other's contact information, but other than that, we were both going in blind. I had heard horror stories about roommates who couldn't get along, but I prayed that I would have better luck.

On move in day, my mom and dad piled into the family van with nearly the entire thing filled with my belongings. Rachel and I loaded up the back seat and trunk of my car so that we could both have room to sit in the front. I remember hardly being able to see out of my rearview mirror because of how high everything was stuffed. When we finally pulled into the parking lot outside of my dorm, Carter Hall, I saw mass chaos. All of the freshman were moving in that day, so there weren't any spots to park, and there was an unloading station that we had to wait in line for. Each building had designated helpers that brought out big, blue bins that made wheeling everything into the dorms a lot easier.

Upon entering my room, I was pleasantly surprised by how spacious it was compared to some of the other rooms I'd seen on college tours. But, my positive impression of the room ended there. Carter had no air conditioning, so within minutes of transporting everything to and from the cars in the August heat, we were all drenched in sweat. There was also no sign of my roommate, Christie.

115

I didn't think much of it because I was too concerned with setting up everything and making my half of the room look cute.

Right before the move in process was scheduled to conclude, in walked Christie. I would later find that punctuality was not her strong suit. Her dad, mom, and toddler brother accompanied her. After we introduced ourselves, I got back to unpacking and let Christie start getting herself situated. Suddenly, I heard her frantically yell, "Tony! Oh my gosh. Put it back! Put it back!"

I looked over to see her two-year-old brother coming out of my closet dragging my extra prosthesis behind him. Christie looked mortified and just stared at me, awaiting my reaction while her mom went to chase Tony, who was now in the hallway with my leg. Instantly, I started busting out laughing.

"I am *so* sorry," she said.

"Are you kidding me? That's hilarious. I bet he'll freak some people out in the hallway."

As soon as she figured out that I wasn't upset, her whole family erupted into a loud guffaw. Christie breathed a sigh of relief, "I think we're gunna get along just fine."

I'm sure she and I have a very different initial meeting story than other roommates, but that moment sealed the deal. We not only just got along, but we would become the best of friends. In fact, our relationship is still running strong 13 years later, both of us having been in each other's weddings. Who would have thought that a good laugh over a leg could be the start of a life-long friendship?

- - -

About a week later, the Toledo Rockets had their first football game. We had a great team, and all the friends that I had just met (mostly from my dorm), decided to go to the game. Even though we weren't old enough to drink, there was alcohol everywhere! The parking lots were all filled with tailgating fans and students. People were so drunk that they just started handing out red solo cups full of beer to anyone passing by. My friends and I did partake, but not much. We were new to campus and were kind of testing the waters, afraid of the threats we heard that undercover police officers were walking around. But, that definitely didn't hold some other people back. While walking to the stadium, someone that I didn't even know approached me from behind.

"Hey, is that a fake leg?" he asked through slurred speech.

"Yeah."

"Duuuude, that's awesome." He now had his arm around my shoulders, probably more for stability than anything. "Can you hide beer in there? We want to sneak some into the stadium." He took a couple cans of beer out of his jeans pockets and tried to hand them to me.

"What?" I asked, confused. "No. It's hollow, but I still have to have room for my leg to go down into it or else I can't walk." I must have looked at him like he was the dumbest person alive. I mean, who asks that?

"Aww, man. Ok." He was genuinely upset and abruptly turned around to walk back to where his friends were standing.

Oddly enough, that wasn't the only time that I got asked to hide beer in my leg. On two other occasions, while at parties, people asked the same question. One even wanted to pour the beer into my leg and then drink out of it. I'm sure people were just trying to be funny, but it's a good example of how some people often don't understand the severity of my situation. Not only were their comments a bit offensive, but pouring beer into my leg would have ruined the interior of my socket. The locking mechanism would have rusted, and it would have cost an exorbitant amount to repair.

Thankfully, I didn't take offense to remarks like these. My mom's advice of thinking about things from other people's perspectives made a lasting impact on me. I know the people who made these types of comments were not trying to upset me. They got a kick out of seeing something different and were trying to have a good time. I could let it upset me, but what good would that do?

When we weren't at parties, my friends and I would go to Windsor, Canada on the weekends to drink and go to the bars because their drinking age was lower. It was only an hour's drive, so to us it was worth the trip. We all had a wild streak that we didn't care to

117

tame. The newfound freedom of being away from our parents really had us pushing limits and doing stupid stuff. It took me about a year or so to reign it in and make better decisions, but I certainly got all my crazy antics out of the way that year.

On one occasion, a big group of my friends, my sister, and one of her friends made the trek up North to Windsor. It was raining heavily, but that didn't bother us too much because the bars and clubs were basically right next to each other; we could go from one to the next without getting totally drenched. But, I was wearing flip flops, and that proved to be a bigger problem. Since I don't have toes to grip the sandal, and the bottom was all wet, it kept falling off. Everyone was dancing, and I couldn't keep up. I thought about taking it off and just holding it, but one look at the dancefloor was enough to deter me. It was covered in shards of glass from broken beer bottles and was doused in puddles of spilled alcohol. About halfway through the night, while at The Treehouse Bar, I was fed up enough to go to the bartender and ask for his help. Typically, I wouldn't do something like that, but I had a little liquid courage helping me out.

"Excuse me, but do you have any duct tape?"

"Whaddya need that for?" he asked. I could just barely see the bottom of his tattoo peeping out from his black concert t-shirt.

I lifted my leg up a bit and pointed to my pink shoe. "My flip flop keeps falling off. I want to tape it to my foot."

He started chuckling, "Well, that's not something you hear every day." I smiled at him flirtatiously, a skill that I learned could get you pretty much whatever you wanted from a guy. "Let me go look for some, ok? But, if I do this, you have to take it off and let me carry it around the bar, ok?"

"I'll tell you what, it's a deal if I get a free shot out of it."

"I can make that happen." He went through some double doors and came back a minute or so later with some clear, packaging tape. "I don't have duct tape, but will this do?"

"Yeah, that should work." I took my prosthesis off and put it on top of the bar as I hoisted myself up onto one of the barstools. He wrapped the tape around my entire foot and shoe about four or five times and then tore the end off. I wriggled it around to see if it was going to hold. Mission accomplished. True to his word, he paraded it around the entire bar, hoisting it into the air like an athlete does his trophy after winning a championship. He got quite the reaction from the crowd. Every girl that I came with started taking pictures of it while dying laughing.

The bartender came back around and handed me my leg. "Well, there's a first time for everything."

"You got that right. Their faces were priceless. Now, how about that shot you promised?" I said, smiling coyly.

Two other friends were up with me at this point, and he was nice enough to make all of us a Buttery Nipple.

When preparing to write this book, I asked my friends if they had any stories or memories that they would share with me in case I might have forgotten a good one. Emily, one of the girls there with me in Windsor that night, mentioned this crazy ordeal. I already had it as a topic that I wanted to include, but what I didn't expect was for her to supply me with the picture that she took of my leg that night. 12 years later and she still had the picture.

- - -

Despite my rowdy and somewhat irresponsible social life, I knew how to reel it in when it came to academics. My grades were important to me, and nothing was going to get in my way of becoming a teacher. When the first day of class came around, I was extremely nervous. I hadn't anticipated how long the walk would take from my dorm to Snyder Hall, where my Introduction to Education class was being held. I thought I left in plenty of time to get there and make a good first impression, but when I got to the doorway of the classroom and peered in, I saw that most of the other students were already in their seats. Of course, the only vacant spots were in the front row. Because I have always been fairly shy around new people, the front row was not an ideal location for blending in the way I'd hoped.

Little did I know, my future husband was sitting in the back with a friend from a neighboring hometown. Having never met him, or anyone else in the class for that matter, I just kept my eyes forward and focused on what the professor was saying. Although I hardly recall any of the details from this day (probably from intentionally trying to block it out of my mind), Bob remembers my entrance like it was yesterday. He recalls me wearing a white skirt and tight, navy-blue top. As soon as he saw me make my late entrance, he turned to his friend and said, "Do you see that girl that just walked in? I'm gunna date her."

At the time, his friend just rolled his eyes and said, "Yeah, ok" with his voice full of skepticism. His friend was already privy to Bob's arrogance, and when we finally had a conversation months later, it didn't take me long to pick up on that trait either.

Although I was wearing a skirt and my prosthesis was clearly visible, Bob doesn't remember noticing it that first day. Maybe the desks blocked his view from the back, or as he says, his "eyes were focused on other things."

My leg might have been overlooked that day, but it only took a couple more weeks for him to notice it. He finally discovered that I was an amputee while at the rec center. It was a place that I frequented religiously. Not only did I work there part-time to get some extra spending money, but it was also where all my friends would hangout. It was right next to my dorm and classes were easy freshman year, so we spent our spare time trying not to gain the freshman fifteen, scope out hot guys, and play all sorts of sports together.

After seeing a flyer hanging in the rec advertising intramural sand volleyball, Christie and I decided to coax our friends from the dorm, John and Troy, into playing on a coed quads team. As soon as we swiped our ID's, we headed through the rec and out the back doors to the sand courts. The other three people on my team sat down on the lawn chairs and took off their shoes. I just stood there, waiting for them to finish so that we could start warming up. You see, sand and I don't get along. Wayne had warned me countless times that going barefoot would cause my rubber foot to deteriorate faster. I imagined that the gritty sand would just expedite that process, so I didn't even think of trying it. I hated being the only one with shoes on, but it was an expensive risk that I wasn't willing to take just so that I could fit in.   In the past, I had even tried playing with only one shoe on, but the height difference threw off my balance. The sand that worked its way into my left shoe would aggravate me to no end, not to mention the discomfort it caused. I couldn't feel the sand in my right shoe, so that was a plus I guess.

As my friends were finishing up getting ready, the other team walked out. Immediately, I knew we were screwed. They were enormous! Christie was 5'2", Troy probably 5'9," John 6' 2", and I was no giant at only 5' 6." Each of their players were at least six inches taller than us.

As we saw them warm up, we started to get an idea of what we were up against. They had perfect form as they warmed up. I assumed that each of them had played high school volleyball. My team, on the other hand, had little to no experience. I was the only one who had played, and I'd just been on the team that one season my freshman year.

The first set went as expected. They killed us! At various points in that set, Christie got hit in the face with the ball as she tried to defend a hard line shot from the other team's tallest player. One whole side of her face was beat read after that. John got his hand caught in the net as he went up to block and basically took the whole net with him as he landed. Then, I dove for a ball, and as I did, piles of sand poured into the top of my prosthesis. After the play ended, I grabbed one of the poles to steady myself, took off my leg, and poured it all out.

Not knowing how else to handle our slaughtering, we decided to do what we did best—make a big joke out of it. Seeing me take my leg off was the last straw for Troy. He bent down, resting his hands on his knees, and just started busting up laughing. After a while, he stood up again and shouted in homage to the famous *Dumb and Dumber* movie, "We got hit in the face, our hands stuck in the net, and now our friends' legs are falling off!"

The other team started dying laughing. "You guys are good sports," one of them said. Despite the loss, we all had a good time. For the next couple months, each time the four of us saw each other, we would repeat what Troy had said during the match: "…our friend's legs are falling off!" We sure got a kick out of it.

After the game ended, Christie and I decided to stay at the rec and get some more exercise since we didn't exactly get the workout we expected during the volleyball game. We swam some laps in the indoor pool for a while and when we tired of that, Christie convinced me to go into the sauna. She loved sitting in there and sweating her butt off. I went along for the ride even though I hated seeing all the half-naked, overweight, old men that always happened to be in there when we were.

I didn't see Bob there that day, but clearly, he was more observant than me because he picked me out of the crowd again. This time, he was even happier to see that I was in a bikini. But, he didn't only have those "typical guy thoughts." He told me, about a year later, that he was so intrigued by me. He stared in awe, just watching me swim and hobble around the pool deck. He was impressed at how much I could do without my leg on and how determined I seemed. Bob didn't work up the courage to talk to me that day, but he knew right then that he wanted to get to know me better. Ironically, my leg is what drew him to me. After all those years of thinking that it would deter guys from wanting to be with me or thinking that I had to overcompensate for it, never had it crossed my mind that my leg would lead someone *to* me.

After a couple more classes together, trying to entice me to his dorm for his mom's banana bread, and convincing me to leave my current boyfriend, we finally started dating the middle of our sophomore year. For the most part, his friends were pretty accepting of me, but he does remember them asking, "Is it weird to date someone with a fake leg?"

"Not really. Your girlfriends all brush their teeth and change into their pajamas before they go to bed. Mine just has one more step. She takes off her leg." It's these types of responses that made me fall for him. He didn't love me despite the fact that I was an amputee; he loved me because I was one.

- - -

Bob wasn't the only one that was openly accepting of my differences while at college. Because of The University of Toledo's size and diverse student population, I fit right in. Since others were quick to embrace me, I too became more accepting. Having come from an upper middle class, suburban area in Ohio, I hadn't really been exposed to racial diversity. College was a different story. There was a big Middle Eastern and African American population that attended. Additionally, I had classes with many physically impaired students as well. One was deaf, one was blind and had a seeing eye dog, and others were in wheelchairs. Not that I was in the majority be any means, but at least I felt like I was represented.

Because people felt more comfortable with me and I with them, I started to take more risks and not care as much about fitting in. I would get a kick out of taking my leg off at parties and showing random people just to see their reaction. I must admit that I loved the attention and liked that my leg gave me a way to stand out as an individual. Everyone kind of has their "thing," and my leg was mine.

Halloween seemed to be the perfect time to put on a show. I decided to be a veteran soldier—more specifically, a Purple Heart recipient. Because many amputees lose limbs while serving in the military, I thought it was pretty realistic. A lot of thought went into my costume. I wore an army green shirt with a camouflage hat, printed out a picture of a purple heart and safety pinned it to my shirt, then secured a toy gun to my belt loop and removed my prosthesis. I rolled up my right pant leg so my entire stump was visible, and even went as far as applying red lipstick to it so that it resembled blood. To complete the costume, I used my spare set of crutches to get around since I didn't have my prosthesis. I was proud of my ensemble, but I wasn't the only one that got a kick out of it.

At the party, it was quite the conversation starter. Most people there had been drinking, so they were brazen and quick to comment. I got a lot of "that's awesome," or "sweet costume" from a bunch of people that I didn't even know. A lot of people, who would normally be too afraid to ask, questioned me about what happened.

Even though it was fun to be in costume, it was also really difficult to maneuver all night while having a beer in my hand. My armpits and hands were throbbing because I wasn't used to using crutches. It gave me a new appreciation for people who have to use them frequently and made me thankful for how well I get around. If I had to guess, I haven't had to use crutches more than 20 days total in my entire life.

Recently, I was at Wright State University's Nutter Center watching my husband's team play volleyball. Bob is the assistant Varsity coach for Bishop Fenwick High School, and his team was playing in the State Semifinals. After the game, I saw a man exiting the stadium wearing a shirt that sported the opposing team's name. He was an above the knee amputee who was not wearing a prosthesis and was using crutches. I got his attention, and we talked for a bit while we both waited for our families to make their way to the exit. He told me a condensed version of his story: His amputation was caused by a necrotic flesh-eating disease that left him in a coma for weeks. When he woke up, he realized his leg had been removed in hopes of stopping the disease from spreading. He had tried prostheses in the past but could never find one that allowed him to walk properly. So, crutches it was.

However, the crutches created a problem of their own. Both of his rotator cuffs were destroyed due to overuse. He admitted that it caused him a great deal of pain. But, even though his story was much more traumatic than mine, I was astounded that he had such a positive outlook about it all. At one point I said to him, "That had to be so hard to wake up and discover that your leg had been amputated. I imagine that took quite the emotional toll on you."

He unexpectedly replied with, "It had to be harder on my wife. She was awake through all of it. I got to miss all of the hard parts." He wasn't bitter or resentful; he was happy he lived through it and was only concerned about his wife.

His amputation took place decades ago, and he's been using crutches every day since. I used them for a day and struggled. I guess people are bound to get used to things, but that day, I saw true strength in that man.

- - -

College wasn't just great for my identity and confidence, but the advancements in prosthetics made a giant leap as well. For starters, I was always told that once I turned 18 and became an adult, I could no longer be a patient at the Shriners Medical Center. But, for a reason unbeknownst to me, they gave Wayne special permission to extend my care until I was 21.

Trips to Kentucky became a bit more difficult because Toledo was even farther away from Lexington, and I was busy with classes. But, when I finally got an opportunity to head that way for a checkup, Wayne had exciting news for me.

He shared that they had just come out with a new skin-type material that could go over my socket to make it look more realistic. He brought in several samples of cosmetic skin covers so that I could pick the color and texture that I wanted. They felt a bit rubbery, but the overall look was very authentic. I will never forget this day. To me, it was the biggest game changer in prosthetics up to this point. The Flex Foot, the locking liner… they were all great, but I couldn't believe that the engineers had finally started to take into consideration the fact that some amputees want an organic-looking, realistic limb. Although there are mixed opinions about the cosmetic look of prostheses in the amputee community, there are some of us who don't want a mechanical, foreign-looking object to be a part of us. I always thought it looked a little too Terminator-like. Knowing that someone out there actually cared about the emotional side of being an amputee really struck a chord with me that day.

With the new skin, I was able to blend in even more. As my self-assurance grew, I no longer tried to hide my leg; instead, I would go out of my way to show it off. I wore shorts and skirts more than ever. Other people noticed the change too. Strangers would come up to me at the mall or other public places, and they would stop me to tell me how realistic it looked or to even congratulate me. I remember an elderly woman coming up to me and saying, "Good for you. You're doing so well. They are making those things look so real today. It's really a wonder what they can do." I had never been prouder to wear a prosthesis in my life.

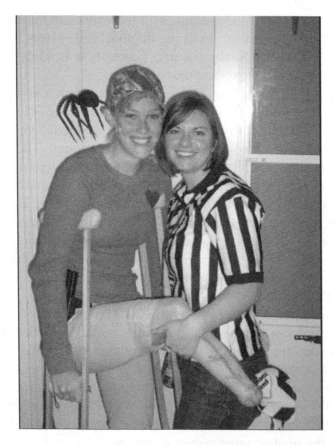

My roommate Christie (Mock) Davis and I at a Halloween party where
I dressed as a Purple Heart recipient.

Chapter 12

Gaining Independence in Adulthood

Only two months after graduating from college, Bob and I got married. We decided to go to Miami, Florida for our honeymoon because of my love of the ocean. We had heard that flying had become quite the process since 9/11, but we both hadn't flown since then. When we showed up at the Cincinnati/Northern Kentucky International Airport the day after our wedding, we were giddy with excitement. Thankfully, we arrived two hours before our departure to ensure we made our flight. We did that as a precautionary thing and didn't think it would actually take that much time, but boy were we wrong.

What we didn't take into account is the fact that I wasn't the "typical traveler." When we showed up to the security area, a TSA agent started barking commands at everyone waiting in line. "Please remove items from your pockets that will set off the metal detector. Take off your shoes and place them in the plastic bins."

I knew my foot, being made of metal, was going to set off the detector. I was used to that because it happened every time I went through one. But, we did as we were instructed, and as we got closer to the front of the line, we started putting our carry-on bags on the conveyor belt so that their machines could scan them. We both took off our shoes as instructed and put them in our plastic, beige bins and sat those on the conveyor belt as well.

Bob went through the metal detector first and got through just fine. However, I tried to avoid the inevitable by telling them what was going to happen before I made a big scene. "I'm going to set it off," I explained.

"What?" the TSA agent asked, clearly not understanding what I was trying to say.

"The metal detector," I tried again. "I'm going to set it off. I have an artificial leg."

"Well, you still need to go through," he stated firmly.

So, of course, the second I stepped through, it started beeping. The light on the top began to flash red. I could feel my face grow warm in embarrassment as I looked around and saw everyone in line staring at me like I was some sort of criminal.

I waited a second to see if he was going to say anything, but when he just stood there and stared at me, I went over to retrieve my bag.

"Ma'am! You cannot touch your belongings!" he authoritatively yelled.

"Oh, sorry," I said, completely caught off guard. "I was just trying to get my stuff." Trying to help, Bob stepped over to collect my things for me.

"Sir! Sir! You cannot touch them either. Leave everything on the conveyor and please step back."

I was now so nervous even though I had done nothing wrong. I couldn't believe how they were treating me. It was like I was guilty until proven innocent just because I had a prosthetic leg.

The TSA agent got on his walkie talkie and said, "I have a code 83 here. Repeat, I have a code 83." Immediately, about five other agents quickly started heading my way. The TSA agent saw them all advancing too and realized his mistake. He got back on the walkie talkie and said, "Correction, I mean a code 23, not 83." The five workers retraced their steps and went back to what they were doing. I don't recall the exact numbers that they used that day, nor do I know what they meant, but it seemed like whatever he said initially was not good. His mistake made me feel even more like a criminal. If I didn't have everyone's attention before, I sure did at that point. All eyes were on me and the line completely stopped moving.

"Please stand right here and spread your legs," he commanded as he escorted me to the side to finally allow other people through the line. He used a hand-held wand and saw that my foot was what made the alarm sound. He then got on his walkie talkie once again and said, "I need a female TSA agent please." He instructed me to sit in a chair and wait for her to come.

When the short, stout female agent came to me, she didn't introduce herself. She just said, "I need you to follow me please. I will take you to a room to better check you in private." I looked at Bob who just shrugged; neither of us knew what to do and figured there wasn't really any other option. I followed her to a small room that had only a couple chairs.

"Please sit down. I need to see your leg. Is there any way you can pull up your pant leg? I need to check for bomb residue or other explosives."

"Sure." I did what I was asked, but all I could think of was *bomb residue*? "People actually put bombs in their legs?" I asked, flabbergasted.

"Well, I'm not really allowed to divulge that information, Ma'am, but we have to take every precaution in order to keep people safe." She took out a white, circular pad that looked like it was made of paper. "Hold out your hands and place them palm up please." She proceeded to wipe the pad on my hands. Then, she wiped it all over my prosthesis, paying special attention to my knee and the interior portion of the socket that she could reach.

After she saw that I was no longer a threat, she told me that I could go on my way and wished me safe travel. I met up with Bob, who was now carrying all my things in addition to his own.

I shook my head and said, "They finally let you hold my stuff?"

"Yeah, they did some kind of special scan of everything."

"Sir, Sir! You cannot touch her things either!" I said, mocking the TSA agent.

"I thought they were going to take you away at one point," he laughed.

"I know, right! How crazy was that? They definitely weren't kidding about increased security. It's no joke."

I was feeling both relieved and a little annoyed at this point. The whole ordeal took us 30 minutes longer than it really needed to. But, with that being said, I completely understand the fact that these types of things need to happen to protect us. I know it was an inconvenience, an embarrassment, and a hassle, but if that's what needed to happen to keep us all safe, then so be it. It just sucked in the moment. And, it wasn't exactly how I envisioned how our honeymoon would start. But, I guess it makes for a good story that we are sure to never forget.

- - -

Flying wasn't the only burden that was placed on me as I grew older. Because I was now 21, I could no longer be considered a Shriners Medical Center patient, which meant I had to start paying for my prosthesis by myself. Thankfully, Wayne was gracious enough to make me two new legs a few months before I turned 21. He hoped that they would last me many years so that I could avoid spending more than was absolutely necessary.

After Wayne handed me those two legs, and I walked out of the medical center's doors for the last time, I never saw him again. In fact, I tried to get in touch with him to write this book but was sadly informed that he passed away in 2016. Not only did some of my history die with him, but I also regret never being able to thank him properly. I expressed my gratitude multiple times as a child, but now that I have a better understanding of his impact, I wish I could have told him again.

Wayne's plan of having two legs helped me get through the next five years without needing another prosthesis. But, I had to find a different prosthetist in order to keep up with routine maintenance. After doing some research and talking to the few amputees that I knew, I narrowed down my choices to Optimus Prosthetics in Vandalia, Ohio. Immediately, I knew I had made the right decision. They were very welcoming, professional, and put the patients' needs first. Although I would always have a special place in my heart for Wayne, my prosthetist at Optimus, Travis Barlow, was very competent and helpful, making him a close second. The nice thing about Optimus is that any routine maintenance is fully covered, and all visits occur without copays. But obviously they need to make their money somehow, so they acquire that upon delivering a new device.

At the time, I was working at Middletown High School in Middletown, Ohio as an English teacher and was covered by Anthem Blue Cross Blue Shield insurance. There were three different plans that I could choose from, but really, there was only one option for me: the top tiered plan that had the highest monthly rate. The other plans would only cover up to $2,500 of a new device, so I would be left to pay over $8,500 out of pocket. Even though it was more expensive per month, it was still advantageous for me because the top plan covered 80 percent of the cost of a new prosthesis.

When the time came for me to get my new device when I was 26, I ended up paying approximately $5,500 after insurance. Even though Bob and I were meticulous in tracking our spending and saved as much as we possibly could, it was still quite the hit to our finances. We were married young at age 21 and 22 years old. We spent a year living in an apartment to save up for a house, drove decade old cars that we paid for in cash, and bought a foreclosure as our first home that needed a ton of work. But, Bob also had $45,000 worth of student loans to pay back. We were able to pay for my prosthesis without any type of payment plan, but that's only because we were so diligent with our savings.

When it was finally time to get a new prosthesis from Optimus Prosthetics, a foot had just come out that allowed amputees to wear high heels. Of course, having spent over a decade battling shoe shopping woes, the adjustable heel height foot was an easy choice. There was a button on the interior side of the prosthesis around the ankle joint that had to be pushed to increase the incline. It had hydraulics and needed to be locked in place when it reached the desired height depending on which heels I wanted to wear. I locked it by pushing the same button on the exterior side of my leg. It would only move about an inch and a half, but finally shoe shopping became something that I enjoyed rather than loathed.

I loved that foot and still use an updated version of it today. Even though it allowed me to wear high heels, I could also wear any other kind of shoe as well. The foot was durable enough for me to work out on too, which meant I only needed one leg instead of two. But, of course the aesthetic improvements didn't come without a cost. The foot alone was about a $3,000 upgrade from my previous one. However, it was an expense that I was willing to pay.

-   -   -

Now that I was an adult, I had to figure out how to navigate my career. I often joked with Bob that I must have the best resume because of how many interviews I landed. However, being a little shy around strangers, my interview skills weren't quite up to par at the beginning of my career. I would interview at these great school districts, and it would come down to one or two other people and me. They *always* chose the other person. In desperation, I finally had to start interviewing at places where I didn't really want to teach. That's how I got my job at Middletown High School. I had heard that Middletown was a difficult school to teach at because its clientele was very diverse and, on average, poor. In fact, when I taught there, 100 percent of the students in the district were on free and reduced lunch. There were often fights in the hallway, kids who were significantly below grade level, and students who were very disrespectful to each other and the staff.

Despite its bad reputation, I had a better connection to those students than any of the other four schools that I taught at. Although it was hard to earn their respect, I found that once I did, they would always have my back. It was a type of loyalty that I hadn't experienced before. They shared more of their personal life with me and were willing to be vulnerable, which lead to a deeper connection. I'm not sure if it was because I liked feeling needed, or if I enjoyed the challenge of trying to get them to succeed. Either way, I loved the fact that I felt like I was making a difference.

But, I didn't just try to help my students academically. I really wanted them to learn life lessons as well. One of the things I focused on was acceptance. Because the school was so diverse, there was some racial tension. There was also a small percentage of the students who were affluent, and there was a bit of a misunderstanding between the "haves" and the "have nots." Students would rarely befriend those who were from the opposite end of the economic spectrum.

The way I tried to tackle all of this was to tell them a very condensed version of what I detail in this book. I wanted them to see me as a person, not just their teacher. Although I remained professional, I have always thought that being open and personal helps the students to relate to me and form a better connection. Once I established that kind of bond, I found it easier to teach them the classroom material; they were more receptive.

Not only did I tell them my story, but I went as far as to take my prosthesis off and show them my stump. I walked without it and showed them the bag of legs that I had acquired over the years. At the end of my little spiel, I allowed them to ask questions.

Before I take my leg off each year, I always warn the students that it might be different or strange to them. I ask if they want to leave the room or close their eyes. About 80 percent are intrigued and eagerly sit on the edge of their seats, 15 percent are skeptical, and there's always a select few that either leave or put their head down. I will never forget one of the star athletes in my class, Zach Edwards, was one of the "select few." Everyone thought of him as this charismatic, big, tough guy, so no one expected that he would ask to leave the room. But, even from the hallway, he peeked his head in occasionally, his curiosity getting the better of him.

Once I finally had it off and started taking questions, one of my former students named Christy asked, "Can I touch your nub?"

"Aww man, you can't ask that. That's weird," said another student in the back.

I just laughed. I thought it was endearing that they cared enough to try not to offend me, but I also got a kick out of the fact that Christy called it a "nub." I'm sure some amputees call their residual limb that, but everyone that I know just calls it their stump. I reassuringly said, "No, it's fine actually. I don't mind. Come on up here. It just feels like normal skin." She made her way up and hesitantly felt the bulbous end of my stump.

"Hey, Mrs. Herber, can I videotape this? I know that sounds weird, but I really wanna show my mom."

"Sure. You're gunna have an interesting conversation when you get home," I joked.

"Can you pass around your leg? I wanna feel it." another student asked.

"Absolutely. How about if you don't want to touch it, you say 'pass' and then just give it to the next person. Ok?" I hobbled over to one of the desks in the front row and gave my student, Emily, my prosthesis. She hesitantly reached out and took it. Just the sight of seeing it in someone else's hands made everyone laugh.

I loved watching their reactions. They got a kick out of me walking on my stump and wiggling it. I heard a lot of "ooo's," "oh man's," and "doesn't that hurt?"

I understand that being this open isn't for everyone. But, I decided a long time ago that I was made like this for a reason. If God designed me this way, He must have wanted me to use it for some type of good. I sure wasn't going to waste an opportunity to spread a little love and acceptance. Because if I didn't, then I was born like this for nothing. And, that was a reality that I couldn't quite accept.

Although my leg demonstrations were fun for most, I did have one student almost pass out and another student actually do so. I guess they thought they could stomach it, but apparently not. I was mid presentation when I saw a girl in the front row start to get a little green. I asked if she was ok, and right as I did, she started to slump over in her chair. The girl beside her caught her before she could go down. Meanwhile, I hobbled over to her and held her steady.

"Someone call the nurse on my phone. Tell her we need help up here."

"Mrs. Herber, no one is answering."

"You've gotta be kidding me! Ok, hang up and call the main office. And, will someone please go get Mr. Williams across the hall. I need his help to move her to the floor."

When Mr. Williams rushed in, I told the students, "Everyone go out into the hallway to give her a little space."

The administration got there, and we were able to give her the help that she needed. I felt terrible that I caused her to have this reaction. In the twelve years that I've been teaching, that was the only time it happened. I don't find it gross or weird because I deal

134

with it every day, so it was a good reminder that others might view it differently.

But, on average, my students respond very well to my leg. I will never forget the time that I brought my backup leg to school so that I could work out after work. My prosthesis was just sitting in a corner of my room by my desk. Two students had already finished their work during study hall, so they were looking for something to keep them occupied. They saw that I had my toes painted on my real leg and on the prosthesis that I was currently wearing, but the toes on my backup leg weren't.

"Mrs. Herber, do you have that toe nail polish with you?" Allie said as she pointed down to my feet.

"Yeah, why?"

"Can Shelley and I paint your toes on your other leg to match?"

"Are you done with your work?" I asked.

"Yeah."

I walked over and picked up my leg so that I could hand it to them. We didn't mean for it to be distracting to the rest of the students in the room, but by this point, everyone was laughing and having a good time with it.

"This is way easier to paint when your leg is off. We don't even have to reach down," Shelley joked.

Although them painting my toes that day seems trivial, it held a lot more weight than it appeared. Not only was my lesson on acceptance sinking in, but students were taking it even further—they were *embracing* me and my differences. The level of comfort that they had with someone that was different than them was what I had always hoped they would achieve.

Acceptance was definitely the lesson that I tried to drive home the most, but I also wanted my students to know that they were capable of overcoming adversity. Whatever I couldn't accomplish in teaching that lesson in the classroom, I tried to do on the court or field. At Middletown, I coached JV softball, freshman girls volleyball, and varsity boys volleyball. Before each season started, the other coaches

135

and I would have our players condition so that they could be more physically fit and perform better in their given sport.

When I played sports in high school, I hated that my coaches would always tell us to run and do all these physical things but would never do it with us. So, now that I was a coach, I vowed to do everything that I told my players to do in hopes of setting a good example. Though, sometimes that was easier said than done. I was very active, so I didn't think keeping up with the kids would be that difficult. But, I was older than them and didn't have quite as much energy. Of course, there was also the obvious—my leg slowed me down a bit. I tried not to let that stop me though. I remember leading a P90x session during boys volleyball conditioning. If you've ever done those workouts, you know how difficult and physically taxing they can be. One of my freshman players in the back row stopped doing the moves and just stood there looking totally defeated.

"Come on, Justin. You've got this," I encouraged.

"No, I most certainly don't. You're killing me back here, Herber!" he dramatically joked. He wasn't trying to talk back or get an attitude; I could tell that he just wasn't used to that intense of a workout. Many of my players hadn't been taught real grit or perseverance. Some of them just didn't have it in them from the get go, but others simply weren't taught those principles at home.

"If you can't do the moves, just modify them. Don't let your feet stop moving though."

"Coach, I seriously can't do this," he said, now starting to whine.

"Ok, you see me up here doing this, right? I'm older than you—"

But before I could finish my sentence, one of the senior captains, Garrett, said, "And she has one leg, dude. So what's your excuse? Come on!" He wasn't really saying it to be mean, but he wanted to hold his teammate accountable and provide some motivation. Although a little unorthodox, it seemed to be effective because when I looked back there, Justin was back at it.

I wasn't one to preach to them or throw my situation in their faces (even though I wanted to sometimes), so I was glad that Garrett did it for me. In most cases, I think quietly leading by example can make a bigger statement, and people tend to respond to it better. But, Garrett was probably right in that particular situation. He knew that that player needed to hear it more forcefully. Justin was a tough one to crack and often gave us quite a bit of push back, but in the end, he made the team and ended up maturing a lot over the years.

Don't get me wrong, those workouts were really challenging for me too. Not only was I winded, but I was so sore after those conditioning days. The only saving grace was that we normally didn't condition two days in a row. Doing it every other day gave my body a much-needed day to recuperate. I never let on to my players how hard it was for me. My pride wouldn't allow that to happen. Moreover, I knew I would lose the whole "lead by example" approach if I gave in to the pain and quit. Hopefully what I did made an impact. If nothing else, it kept me in shape.

-   -   -

Not only did my students and players learn to accept me, but my coworkers did as well. Middletown High School and Lakota West High School (where I now teach) are very large districts. It was quite common to not know other teachers by name in staff meetings or in the teacher's lounge. If one of my friends was talking to a coworker who didn't know who I was, they would simply say, "You know, the one with the fake leg." They would immediately respond with, "Oh, yeah, I know who you're talking about."

I was always conditioning with my players in the hallway, so my leg was hard to miss. Plus, students talk... a lot. When I showed my students my leg, they would talk about it all day. Many teachers would come up to me and ask if what the kids were saying was true. Most of them were shocked that I would start off the year being so vulnerable and personal.

But, they would soon find out that I wasn't just vulnerable with my students; I was open about my leg with them as well. One of the best examples of this occurred at our staff Christmas party one year.

A couple weeks before the party, the host set the ground rules for the white elephant gift exchange that we would be having: it was supposed to be funny and cost no more than $15. After seeing the movie, A Christmas Story, I got the idea to make a homemade present. Not just any present—a lamp leg. I got my extra prosthesis out of the closet and put a red, shiny high heel on my foot. I spent about an hour trying to affix the shade to the top part of my leg. We didn't have any extra lamp shades lying around, so I took the one off my living room lamp.

I was proud with how it turned out, but disguising it proved to be equally as challenging as constructing the leg itself. I placed it in an oversized gift bag and put another one upside down on top of it. I had to bear hug it just to carry it. With it being my first year at Lakota and only having spent a couple months with these people, I hoped that they would play along and see the humor in it.

Upon entering my coworker's house , I immediately started to get stares and questions.

"Did you bring a dead body in there, Kendra?" one of my outspoken coworkers named Jason asked.

"Oh, just wait," I replied, grinning from ear to ear. I sat it under the Christmas tree and mingled with everyone until it was time for the gift exchange to start.

We all sat in a circle on the floor with the presents in a pile in the center. The first person chose a gift and then proceeded to open it. The next person in the circle could either steal a present that had already been opened or they could open a new one. The gifts ranged from nice, thoughtful gifts like a dream catcher to gag gifts that no one really knew what they were.

The woman who opened the lamp leg was named Jeni. She's our school's secretary. Everyone that works at Lakota knows that the school would fall apart if it wasn't for her. But, she's also fiery and has a great sense of humor. I couldn't have picked a better person to open my gift; I knew she would appreciate my handiwork.

I will never forget the look on her face when she took the top bag off the leg. She started dying laughing and said, "Well, I guess there's no question to who brought this one."

Being a little timid around big crowds, I felt myself get nervous. But, knowing that bringing that type of present couldn't warrant a reticent response, I said, "Now, Jeni, you know I'm gunna have to have that back at the end of the party, right?"

"What the hell? What kind of gift is that?" joked Jason. "Indian giver!"

"Whatever. You're just jealous you didn't get it."

"Yeah, you caught me."

The next year when I didn't show up at the Christmas party with a gift for the exchange, someone asked, "You're not participating this year?"

"Nah. I'm not sure how I could top my last year's gift, so I'm not even going to try."

- - -

Only a couple months later, the same coworker from the Christmas party called my classroom phone. I was in the middle of a lesson, but I stopped to answer it.

"Hello," I said.

"Hey, it's Jason. I have a strange request."

"Oh gosh. That's scary coming from you. But, go ahead. Ask away."

"Did you happen to bring your spare leg to school today?" I could tell from his voice that he was trying to keep a straight face on the other end of the phone.

"Yeah, why?" I asked.

"Can my students borrow it for this class period?"

"Well, I guess that depends. What are they gunna do with it?"

"We're studying WWI and trench warfare. They're giving a presentation and would love to use it as a visual aid."

"Are you being serious? I know you're always joking, but this time I can't tell if you're for real."

"I actually am this time. Can I send one of them up to your room so that they can get your leg?"

"Sure," I said. "Take good care of that thing; it's expensive," I joked.

I was glad that they all knew I didn't take myself (or my situation) too seriously. My prosthesis has a tendency to break social barriers and even gives people cause to laugh on occasion.

Over the years, my coworkers have responded similarly to my students; they are always accepting and politely roll with the punches (even when I throw a crazy curve ball at them, or them at me). My work environment would be a lot different if that wasn't the case. I'm glad I work in a place where I can be comfortable being myself.

Chapter 13

My Pregnancy Saga

Pregnancy and childbirth are difficult for any woman, but many people don't realize the added issues that some amputees have to deal with when it comes to that stage of life. Swelling and weight gain alter the fit of amputee's prostheses and oftentimes makes it extremely uncomfortable or painful to wear them. Sarah Peterson, an author with the Amputee Coalition, interviewed a few women right after they gave birth. One of them gave some comical (but accurate) advice to other amputees who are going through the post-partum process: "Be sure to use crutches because you'll wet your pants if you try to hop." Although I am I aware of these complications now, I hadn't given any thought to what I was getting myself into when Bob and I decided to start trying for a baby.

We'd been married for five years at that point and were finally ready to give parenthood a whirl. But, as a lot of couples do, we struggled to get pregnant. Bob always remained hopeful and confident that it would eventually happen, but I wasn't so sure. I found myself getting jealous and bitter when I saw all the birth announcements on Facebook and the women at church with their cute baby bumps.

Thankfully, a year and a half later, I finally had a healthy pregnancy, which made all the waiting worth it. During my first trimester, I had a routine checkup at Optimus Prosthetics. I excitedly told my prosthetist, Travis, about the pregnancy and shared some of my concerns.

"What is going to happen when I start gaining weight? You've told me before that I shouldn't gain or lose more than 5-10 pounds if I want my leg to fit. But, my OB says that I should gain 30."

"Well, I've actually never had a patient who is pregnant before. So, this will be a first for both of us. I want to be upfront with you, though. From what my coworkers have said, they've never had a patient go full term without being in a wheelchair. I know you're not accustomed to that, but you might want to prepare yourself if in fact that needs to happen," Travis said.

"A wheelchair? Really?" I asked, deflated.

"Yeah. Crutches aren't an option during pregnancy because of the risk of falling. We wouldn't want anything to happen to the baby."

"That makes sense. I just didn't realize it would be an issue. Maybe I'll be the first who doesn't have to do that."

I had a lot of trouble gaining weight during my first trimester because I was so nauseous. At my twelve-week checkup, I actually got scolded for it.

"Go ahead and step up on the scale, Kendra," my nurse instructed. I removed my shoes and did as I was told. "136. You've only gained one pound this entire trimester." She said it more as a question than a statement. "You really need to make sure you're gaining enough weight so that your baby gets all the nutrients it needs," the nurse continued.

"Well, I'm trying, but it seems like every time I look at food, I vomit. Trust me, I love food. I'd be eating it if I could," I tried to joke. "I keep a Tupperware container in my car and puke in it as I'm driving to work most mornings. The other day I puked in the bushes as I was making my way into the building. There are some days that I can't even teach my class. I get to work and sit in the teacher's lounge while another teacher covers for me." The words just started rolling out of my mouth. Apparently, I didn't know how badly I needed to vent. The pregnancy hormones were in full force, and it was all I could do to keep myself from crying.

The nurse seemed to soften up a bit after hearing that and stopped lecturing me. "I'm so sorry, sweetie. We'll get you past this. The first trimester can be tough on a lot of women," she said sympathetically. "You're taking a prenatal vitamin, right?" she asked.

"Yeah, but I'm afraid the baby isn't really getting any benefit from it because I can never keep it down."

"Wow, you must have a really sensitive stomach. Have you tried Flintstone Complete vitamins?"

"The chewable ones? Yeah, but not since I was a kid," I said, laughing. "Why?"

"They are almost just as good as prenatals, but they're easier on the stomach. Why don't you try those instead? We will also get you some Zofran to help with the nausea. You put one little pill under your tongue, and it will dissolve," the nurse instructed.

The Zofran and Flintstone vitamins were a big help, but I still found that if I let myself get even remotely hungry, I would vomit. I kept a bag of dry cereal on my nightstand so that I could have a handful every time I woke up during the night. Bob *loathed* this process because the bag inside of the box would rustle with every single handful I got out. Heaven forbid *his* sleep get interrupted.

When I got to thirty weeks, I started getting cocky and thought I wasn't going to have an issue with my socket fitting. However, with the third trimester came an insatiable hunger. I would pack snacks everywhere; I had carrots in my purse, pretzels in my car, and a whole box of Cheez-its in my classroom. Needless to say, I finally started putting on weight. Thankfully, it was all in my stomach, so my leg was still fitting fine.

However, two weeks later, in the dead of summer, the heat started getting to me. Of course, the only parts of my body that swelled were my foot and stump. I did everything that I could to counteract it. Removing my two stump socks that I wore over top of my liner made a world of difference. That change alone got rid of ¼ inch of bulk around the whole circumference. The silicone liner helped to combat the swelling because of its tight fit. However, as soon as I took it off to relax for the evening, my stump would blow up like a balloon.

Because I was on my feet all day, my stump would start to throb, and I would get the feeling that it was falling asleep. The tingly feeling was very painful, and it took everything that I had to not grimace when I walked. The only one that I would let see my pain is my husband. Bob patiently waited on me while I sat on the couch with my leg elevated. He massaged my stump until I would take my shower before bed. I learned the hard way that taking a warm shower in the morning made it almost impossible to even fit my stump in my prosthesis because of how much it would swell. The few times that I was able to stuff it in, I ended up taking my prosthesis off within minutes. Upon removal, I saw that my entire leg was beat red and hot to the touch. Blood couldn't circulate properly.

I would often have to hold Bob's hand to hobble around without my leg on in the evenings, which I never had to do before being pregnant. The extra weight that I carried put too much pressure on my thin stump.

One day, mid-way through my third trimester, Bob came into our bedroom and said, "Don't be mad, but I got you something."

"Oh gosh. What'd ya do?" I said, playfully rolling my eyes.

"I got you a pedicure."

"Oh no," I said, completely failing at hiding my disappointment. "Bob, you know how awkward that's going to be!"

"No, I already talked to them about it. They'll give you half off since they're only doing one foot."

"Oh my gosh. That's so embarrassing."

"Come on. That's a great deal, and you really deserve it. You were just saying the other day that you can't even bend down and touch your toes because of your belly. Let me do this for you."

I finally relented and begrudgingly must admit that I'm glad I did. However, the language barrier between the nail tech and I made the process a bit challenging.

After she ran the warm water in the basin so that my feet could soak, she motioned for me to put them in. I, of course, only put my left foot in. She tapped my prosthetic foot and then pointed to the water.

"Oh, I'm sorry, but my foot isn't allowed to get wet. You'll just be doing this one," I said, pointing to the foot that was already submerged. I knew as soon as I said it that she didn't understand. So, I started using more arm motions and finally conveyed my message.

By the time my nails were ready to paint, another nail tech had made her way over with a client that sat down right beside me.

The two nail techs spoke back and forth for a minute or so and then the other one asked me, "Do you want her to paint your other foot so that it will match? It will be no charge."

"Oh, yeah, that'd be great. Thank you. I bet this is her first time painting fake toes," I joked.

She relayed the information back to my nail tech, and she grinned from ear to ear while nodding her head yes.

"Well, this is a first for me too."

Although it was a bit awkward at first, the fact that my nail tech was such a good sport really added to the relaxing experience.

-   -   -

Despite everyone's initial thoughts, I did make it through the whole pregnancy without having to use a wheelchair. At 39 weeks, I thought that my water was starting to leak a little, so Bob and I gathered up our bags and headed to the labor and delivery section at Kettering Hospital in Dayton, Ohio. The nurses hooked me up to a machine to monitor my contractions and another to track the baby's heart rate. As soon as the heart rate monitor was set up, the nurse looked at Bob and said, "Um, sir, can you please push that red button on the wall behind you?"

I vividly remember the exact words he said in return: "Red is bad." What seemed like the emergency crew came rushing into the room. "What's going on?" Bob asked.

"We can't find the baby's heart rate."

"At all?!" I asked.

"Nope, not for the last three minutes." My heart sank. Somehow, I didn't cry. I think I was too shocked. For a few horrible minutes, I thought we had lost her.

Another nurse adjusted the heart rate monitor and said, "Ok, that's better. Everything seemed fine now."

Only about five minutes after that, she told us that my water wasn't leaking and that I could go home if I wanted.

"Whoa, one minute you're telling me you can't find a heart rate and the next you say go home?"

Bob, being the more persistent of the two of us stepped in and said, "Yeah, we're not leaving. She only has a week left. You can at least monitor the baby awhile longer to see if everything is ok."

"I completely understand. I'm going to talk to the doctor and see what I can do to get you induced.

14 hours later, my water had been broken, and I'd been induced, but I still wasn't progressing. Every single time I laid on my left side, my baby's heart rate decelerated. I had to lay on my right side the entire time, and I was so sore and uncomfortable. I also hadn't eaten in almost 24 hours. And, if people know me even a little bit, they know how big of a deal that is. I eat all. the. time.

At 11:00 a.m., they finally decided to do a c-section. "Do you want to take off your prosthesis?" the nurse asked.

"I don't know. Should I?" Not only did I not know what I was doing or what to expect because it was my first child, but I was also exhausted, in pain, and nervous.

"Well, it might get pretty dirty. Let's play it safe and just remove it."

A nurse's aide came to roll me to the operating room. I had a blanket over my legs, and I guess she didn't get the memo that I was an amputee. She stopped rolling the bed about thirty feet before the operating room doors. "Go ahead and get down. You can walk right through those doors," she said.

I took the blanket off and hopped down from the bed. Immediately, I could see the terror on her face.

"Oh my gosh! No one told me you were an amputee. I am so sorry. I should have rolled you into the room. Do you want to get back on the bed?"

I laughed at her reaction. I bet she didn't have that happen too often. "No, it's not far. I'm fine." I hobbled into the operating room and hoisted myself up onto the table where the anesthesiologist was waiting for me.

The OB went about her business and a short seven minutes later, my firstborn, Gabriella, came into the world. But, everything was eerily silent.

"Why isn't she crying?" I asked Bob.

146

"I have no idea. I'll ask."

"Dad, do you want to hold her?" asked the nurse. At that very moment, Gabriella started wailing.

"Oh, everything is ok?" Bob asked, relieved.

"Yeah, the cord was wrapped around her neck and c-section babies normally don't cry right away because their lungs aren't squeezed when going through the birth canal. We had to suck out the fluid, and now she's just fine. You have a perfectly healthy baby."

Relief washed over both of us. Knowing that c-section babies don't cry right away would have been more helpful than my two-day childbirth class that barely mentioned c-sections at all.

Hearing that my baby was completely normal was surprising to me for some reason. Sure, the ultrasounds never showed any problems, but I had always had it in the back of my mind that God might give me a child with some sort of special needs because I would likely be more understanding of a baby who required more attention or care. I was also worried that my birth defect might be genetic. But, that wasn't the case. Even though my nurses never said it exactly, my daughter had 10 fingers and 10 toes. She wasn't like me. I know better than anyone that she would have been completely fine if she were like me, but I couldn't help but to be relieved.

I certainly was grateful that she didn't need any extra care because having a major surgery and taking care of a newborn baby while being an amputee was probably the most challenging thing I have ever done. Bob had to change all the diapers at the hospital since it was hard for me to even get out of bed.

When I went home, things got harder. On top of everything women who undergo a c-section have to endure, I also had a prosthesis to put on in the middle of the night in order to get up and feed my baby. The adjustable hospital bed made it easier for me to get out of the bed, but at home, I had no such luxury. My incision hurt so bad when I bent my torso. The first night that I was home, it was hard enough to get myself up to a sitting position in bed, but from there, I still had to bend over and put my liner, socks, and prosthesis on. By the end of the ordeal, I was in tears. I'm sure some of that was due to all the post-delivery hormones, but I still remember the

147

pain to this day. Bob, being a sound sleeper, slept through the whole thing. I'm not sure why I was so stubborn and didn't ask him for help, but I was a new mom and had something to prove I guess.

The next night didn't go much better. This time I tried to avoid the pain by not putting my leg on during the nighttime feeds. I hobbled around changing Gabriella's diaper, pumping, bottle feeding, and rocking her to sleep. I had just about finished with my hour-long routine and gotten her to sleep when she pooped and I had to basically start the process all over again. Not only was I exhausted and frustrated, but I was physically tired too. Walking around without my leg on added a whole other challenge. At that point, I decided to call in reinforcements. Bob had to get up for work in only a few short hours, so I picked up my cell phone and called my mother-in-law, Sonya, who was sleeping in our guest room upstairs. I could hear her phone ring and felt silly for calling someone who was so close in proximity, but the doctors told me I wasn't allowed to go up the stairs until my incision healed. Thankfully, Sonya had volunteered to stay with us for a week to give Bob and I some extra help during the acclimation period. Before we went to sleep each night, she told me to call her if I needed anything, and boy did I ever.

I gave her the rundown on what I had already done and what I wanted her to do. I handed Gabriella to her, feeling the same relief when a runner passes the baton in a race. Practically as soon as my head hit the pillow, I was sound asleep.

- - -

For a while, I went about motherhood as most women do. My disability didn't really come into play again until my daughter was about a year old. Since Bob was coaching volleyball and had practice one afternoon in August, I decided to take Gabriella to the pool. It had a zero-entry section that was great for her since she had recently just started walking. But, anything water-related is always more complicated for me than most, and the day did not go as I had hoped. When we got home from the pool, Bob was already home

148

from practice. I immediately started venting to him about the events from that day.

"I am never taking her to the pool by myself again!" I told Bob as I came in the door.

"Uh, hi to you too," he said, only half joking.

"I'm sorry. I just had the worst day."

"Why? What happened?"

"Well, first, the pool was crowded and the only chair available was, of course, the furthest one away from where you get in. I had to set my leg on the chair, pick up Gabriella, and hobble all the way over to the zero-entry area. You know how rough that concrete is. It killed my stump!"

"Why didn't you just set your leg down closer to the pool? No one would have cared," said Bob. Bob, like a lot of men, is a "fixer." He is always trying to fix the problem, when I'd rather him just listen.

"Wouldn't you freak out if some random person's leg was next to your stuff? No, that was not an option. Plus, I had to make sure it didn't get wet."

"True."

I barely paused for him to comment. I was on a roll now and continued, "And, your lovely daughter here decided it would be a great idea to keep getting out of the water and running away. I didn't think about her being able to walk now. With my leg off, I couldn't keep up with her. It was super dangerous. She wouldn't just sit in the zero-entry part anymore. All she wanted to do was go go go."

"Oh man, I didn't think about that either," he said sympathetically. "It's no big deal. I'll go with you next time, and I can chase her."

"But it *is* a big deal. I want to be able to take my daughter to the pool. I ended up having to hold her in the deeper water, but then I was bouncing around on my left leg the whole time, which got super tiring."

"I'm sorry things didn't go well. Remember that this will only last for a little bit. Once she gets older, she will understand that she can't run off. In the meantime, I'll go with you, ok?"

"I guess that will have to work. It just sucks that I have to wait for a day that you can go now. I want to just be able to go with her whenever I want."

Bob brought me in for a hug. Because he knew me so well, he understood that half of the issue was the fact that I had to admit to myself that I couldn't do what everyone else could, and that's always been a tough pill for me to swallow. Why should a leg get in the way of me caring for my child? I wanted to be superwoman and do it all. Plus, I had something to prove: I needed people to see that amputees can do these things. But, I couldn't that day. And although I knew that *I* wasn't a failure, I couldn't help but be frustrated *by* my failure.

-   -   -

Shortly after the pool incident, when Gabriella was about 14 or 15 months old, we encountered another unforeseen issue. I was just sitting down on our area rug in the living room after having cleaned up the dinner mess to play with Gabriella. Normally, I took off my leg at that point in the evening to be more comfortable after a long day. I pushed the button to release my leg, but before I could start rolling down the liner to take that off too, I heard Gabriella start to scream. Tears were streaming down her face as she ran as far from me as possible.

Bob was just coming into the room and said, "What's all this about?"

"I have no idea. She just started screaming and ran away."

"Huh. That's weird. Come here, sweetie," Bob said to Gabriella. He picked her up, and she started to calm down. Then, he carried her back to the living room where I was. As soon as he sat her down by me, she started screaming all over again.

"Oh my gosh. I think she's scared of my leg."

"Really? She's never been scared before," said Bob.

"Maybe she is finally old enough to understand that I'm taking off a part of my body. That would be pretty creepy. I bet she thinks a part of her might come off." I looked at Gabriella and said, "It's ok, sweets. Momma isn't hurt. Come here."

150

She stood right where she was, frozen in fear. I picked up my prosthesis and showed it to her. "You can touch it. It won't hurt you."

"No no!" she said as she started to cry again.

Completely crushed, I looked at Bob. "What do we do?"

"I don't know. She'll get used to it though... just give her some time. What happens if you put it back on?

I thought Gabriella would continue to be scared of me, but as soon as it was back on, she came right over and sat in my lap.

"I will not have my daughter afraid of me," I told Bob. "I'm going to figure something out."

The very next day, I took a whole pack of stickers out of the closet and sat back on the floor with Gabriella. She was obsessed with stickers at the time, so I figured I would use what she loved to get her to change her mind about my leg. I started off by just having her put them on my prosthesis while it was on. I didn't want to rush into anything.

After Gabriella got comfortable with that, I slowly started to take my leg half off while she was putting the stickers on. Sure enough, her fear dissipated. By the end of the week, I could leave my prosthesis lying in the middle of the room and walk around on my stump without her even caring. Bob just smiled at the two of us. I could tell he thought my idea was pretty genius.

When I had my second daughter, Eliza, we encountered the same exact phenomenon. Children's developmental stages are so fascinating. At almost precisely the same age, Eliza started exhibiting the same behavior—the crying, the running away, the fear. So, I went back to my bag of tricks and stuck with what worked with Gabriella. Sure enough, the sticker method succeeded again. This time was a bit easier because I had Gabriella's help. She would get on the floor with me and touch my leg, showing Eliza that it was ok. Because she wanted to do everything her big sister did, she followed suit not too long after.

- - -

Much like my mom did many years ago, I try to follow in her footsteps and educate others (especially children) about what makes me different. It has really seemed to rub off on my kids, who are more accepting than most children their age. We've had too many conversations to count about the fact that God made me special; celebrating our differences is a norm in our household.

I knew it was inevitable that one day my kids would have to answer the question that I have had to my entire life: What happened to your mom's leg? When Gabriella was about three, her friends at daycare would gravitate to me when I picked her up. Sometimes they would actually touch my prosthesis out of curiosity. I hadn't exactly prepped Gabriella on what to say when someone asked, so I was kind of caught off guard when I heard it asked of her.

I couldn't have been prouder of the response she gave them: "Oh, that's just her special leg." She said it so matter-of-factly. She left it at that too, because to her, there was no other explanation needed. The child who asked was satisfied with the answer, and we both went out of the door.

Her classmates became more perceptive as they got older, so Gabriella and I got asked more and more questions. She never grew impatient or became annoyed. I could tell she actually liked answering them. One afternoon, after being asked yet another question, I had an idea.

"Gabriella, what do you think about me coming to talk to your class about my leg?"

"Yeah!" she said enthusiastically.

"Do you think your friends would like that? I think it would help explain a little more about my leg.

"Sure, Momma. When are you going to come?"

"Well, I need to talk to your teacher first and see if it's ok."

Gabriella's teacher and the director both jumped at the opportunity to have me as their guest speaker. They thought the kids could really benefit from learning about someone who was different from them so that they might be more accepting of others.

I knew I would have to take a different approach to my normal spiel that I give. High schoolers aren't exactly the same as four-year-olds. I decided not to take my leg off in fear of scaring the kids. Instead, I planned to bring in my first prosthesis from when I was two. I thought they might get a kick out of how small it was. I also bought a book that I could read to them titled "My Dad the Superhero." The book is about a kid named Milo that brings his dad in for show and tell. He is so excited to tell his classmates about his dad's "magic leg."

When I got to the school to share my story, the director asked if it would be ok to bring out all the kids. After telling her "the more the merrier," kids started lining up to come out into the lobby. The book was a hit. They loved all the talk about superheroes. The more I talked, the more comfortable they became. By the end, they were asking to touch my prosthesis, telling me their own stories of what makes them different, and making connections to the characters in the book.

When I asked if they had any questions, one kid's hand shot into the air. "I play soccer too!"

Gabriella's teacher, Miss Alex, looked at me and we both chuckled. "Well, that's not exactly a question. Does anyone have a *question* for Mrs. Herber...about her *leg*?" she asked.

"I do. I do!" said a little girl with blonde, spiral curls. "One time, I saw a guitar."

"That's neat," I said, not knowing entirely how to respond. I don't know how elementary teachers do it. There's definitely a reason I teach high school.

Who knows if I made any impact on those kids that day, but hopefully I at least planted a seed about how to treat people who are different. I know that it made an impression on Gabriella that day because just the other night, when Bob and I were getting her ready for bed, she pulled "My Dad the Superhero" off her bookshelf and asked to read it to me. She's one of the few five-year-olds that knows how to read and pronounce the word prosthesis. After she read it, she looked up at me and said, "Momma, I wanted to read you this book because it's not how you look that matters. It's what's in your heart." I'm not a very emotional person, but I would be lying if I said I didn't have tears that came to my eyes during that moment. She understands more about love and acceptance than some adults. She gets it.

Chapter 14

Personal Achievements

Despite some of the challenges that I've encountered in my life, I've accomplished a lot. That's not to say that any of my big, physical accomplishments were easy. In fact, I have more pride because they weren't.

My sophomore year of college my sister really wanted to run a 5k. She knew that training for the race would keep her active and healthy. But apparently signing herself up wasn't enough.

"You'll do it with me then, right?" Rachel asked.

"You know I hate running."

"I know, but we'll be like accountability partners. We can help each other stay on track."

"I can barely run a mile, Rache. You know that, right?"

"But we have months to get ready. You're in killer shape. You'll be fine."

"I might be in decent shape, but you know running is different. I'm not in *that* kind of shape."

"So... you'll do it?" Rachel asked persistently.

"Ugh." I said, rolling my eyes. "I guess so, but I'm not going to be setting any records. My goal is to just finish without having to stop and walk."

For the next few months, I ran two or three times a week while still doing my other workouts in between. It was difficult at first, but like anything, it got easier the more I did it. I know so many people that love running. I just can't relate on any level. I hate every single aspect of it—how mundane it is, the fact that my legs itch/tingle, and the way it makes me feel like I'm breathing through a straw. Don't get me wrong, I love exercising, but I find no joy in running. I thought it might grow on me once I competed, but I was wrong.

After months of training, I wasn't exactly confident in my ability, but I thought finishing the race without stopping would be a breeze. I had run three miles plenty of times over the last few months and had no reason to believe I couldn't do it on the day of the race.

I left Toledo after classes on Friday afternoon to go back home. The race was being held at my church in Tipp City, Ohio the following day. Bob decided to make the trip with me so that he could be there for moral support.

"Aren't you going to eat anything?" I asked Rachel the next morning as I drank a glass of orange juice and ate a light breakfast.

"Nope. I don't want it to weigh me down. I'll get something after."

"Ok, but it'd probably give you more energy."

"Oh, so now you know everything about running, huh?" she joked. "Bob, are you sure you don't want to run with us? I bet you could still register when we get there."

"Ha, good one. I only run if someone's chasing me. I'll wait for you guys at the finish line," he said as he wolfed down a bowl of cereal that could have fed three people.

When we got to the church, the parking lot was full of cars and people walking around with numbers on their shirts.

"Come on, let's go sign in," said Rachel.

I followed her over to the registration table and told the person my name. He handed me some safety pins to help secure the number to my shirt and then pointed me in the direction of the starting line. People were already lined up, chomping at the bit like they'd win some kind of medal for crossing the *starting* line first.

"I'm not about to go up there with those people," I told Rachel.

"No kidding. They'll run us over with how slow we are. Let's stay closer to the middle."

I glanced over my shoulder to scope out who was behind us. They were clearly the walkers. They had strollers and didn't seem to have a care in the world.

"Yup, these are our people," I joked.

Suddenly, there was a gun that fired, and everyone was off. The first mile was fairly easy. My training seemed to have paid off. But, shortly thereafter, I could tell I was getting winded.

"What's up with all these hills?" I asked. "I totally didn't plan for this." The track at the rec center was obviously flat as a pancake, and it had never dawned on me that I should increase the incline when I practiced on the treadmill.

"You got this," Rachel encouraged. So, I pressed on, determined not to stop running. Around the start of the second mile, my stomach started to churn. For all the same reasons mentioned earlier, my body had to work harder to compensate for the lost energy. I could feel myself start to overheat.

"My cheeks are beet red, aren't they?" I asked her, completely out of breath.

"Uh, just a tad," Rachel joked. I knew the answer before I even asked because they felt like they were on fire. For some reason, I don't sweat much, so I'm much more prone to overheating. Normally I would just take a break if I felt it coming on, but I wanted to meet my goal of not having to stop. I pressed on. But, after only a minute or two, I stopped dead in my tracks and hurled all over the grass right next to me.

As if that wasn't embarrassing enough, an old man that was probably in his seventies came up beside me, put his arm around me, and said, "You can do it! I'll run by you so we can do this together." He was so sweet, but I was quite ashamed that a man 50 years my senior was doing better than me.

I looked over at Rachel. I could see that she felt bad for me but tried to lighten the mood by saying, "Come on! Puke and rally!"

"Puke and rally," I repeated, hoping for it to become my mantra. I willed my feet to keep going. The pause to throw up only took about ten seconds. Surprisingly, I didn't have to stop to get sick or take a break for the rest of the race. When the finish line came into view, I got my second wind and started running as fast as I could even though my legs felt like jello. Rachel picked up speed next to me as well.

After we crossed the line with big smiles on our faces, I looked over at her and said, "We totally aren't counting my puke break as me stopping, are we?"

"No, of course not. But, I may have to tell people about it," she said in jest.

"Oh, huh uh. You don't get to tell *my* story. I can't wait to see the look on Bob's face when I tell him I puked mid race."

We both got a good laugh out of it to say the least. I would like to say that I've run many races since then and that I got progressively better and ran even further, but that would be a lie. In fact, I haven't run another race since. I *still* hate it. However, I now have the pride of saying that I did it… and that's enough. To me, it's just like watching the same movie twice; there's really no point because I already know what is going to happen. Running another race wouldn't be twice as magical; it would be even worse because I know just how bad it would be before starting.

-   -   -

In addition to running my first and only 5K, I tackled another feat around the age of 25. Christie, my roommate from college, moved out to Phoenix, Arizona to work at the VA hospital for her pharmacy residency. Bob and I explored the city while Christie was at work, but during the evenings and on the weekend she served as our tour guide. She had us doing all sorts of fun things, one of which was climbing Camelback mountain. The unique thing about that particular mountain is that it's right in the city. And, as its name suggests, it's shaped exactly like a camel's back.

Before we set out to climb it, I had no qualms whatsoever (partially because mountains never appear that big when you're looking at them from far away). Phoenix in February is gorgeous, the sunny, 75-degree weather making it just about perfect for outdoor activities. My mind was too focused on how awesome the warm sun felt compared to the bitter cold back home to think about how difficult the climb would be.

I had been on a lot of hikes in my life, but I'd never climbed a mountain. Camelback is right around 2,700 ft. in elevation. I was completely ignorant as to whether or not that was considered tall. All

I knew was that Christie brought her dog with her, so I assumed it couldn't be too bad.

The beginning was pretty leisurely, but as we ascended, it got more difficult. There were a few spots where we had to use hand holds to hoist ourselves up. At the top of the lower of the two humps, my legs felt rubbery. I looked at Bob and said, "I don't think I can do this. Why don't you and Christie keep going. This is a really good spot to sit and wait for you guys." He looked around and saw that I was right. There was a wide open, flat area that a lot of people used to take the same break that I was wanting to.

"Nope, absolutely not. You're not coming all this way without getting to the top. We can take as many breaks as you want, but you're doing this. Imagine how proud you'll be of yourself when you're done."

"Yeah, but I still have to go all the way down once I get up there. I'm not even half of the way done, and I don't want to get to a point where I can't go on."

"Nope, you're not stopping. I won't let you," he said matter-of-factly. This may make Bob sound controlling or insensitive, but he's not at all. I know what his intentions were and how big of a heart he has. His ability to push me to be a better person in practically all facets of my life is probably the number one thing that drew me to him in the first place. I wanted to be frustrated with his persistence, but I knew he was right. So, just like the race, I pressed on.

After only a few short breaks, we reached the summit. Christie, Bob, and I sat down, dangling our feet over the edge while Christie's dog, Roxy, downed an entire bowl of water. The view was stunning. The green trees stood out against the brown dirt. I was so used to seeing grass in Ohio, but there was hardly any in Arizona. I could see the main highway that goes through Phoenix and a bunch of other smaller mountains. While taking in my surroundings, I was already glad that I didn't stop before reaching the peak.

We stayed up there for about 15 minutes, taking a much-needed rest. As soon as I stood up to make my descent, I knew it was going to be rough. This was nothing like running. I never once got out of breath. Cardiovascularly speaking, I was fine, but my leg muscles kept telling my brain to stop. About a quarter of the way down, I started having trouble lifting my right leg high enough to clear the rocks and other obstacles along the path. Hindsight being 20/20, I should have taken another break, but my competitive nature paired with my stubbornness and pride made me press on.

I was looking straight ahead, so I had no idea what made me fall, but I could feel the vibration of my prosthetic foot hitting something. Before I had time to react, I dropped like a ton of bricks. That probably wouldn't have been that bad, but I hit my tailbone right on the edge of a rock. Immediately, tears welled up in my eyes. I tried to be tough, but my lip started to quiver. Bob could tell right away that I was hurt.

"Are you ok?" he asked.

"That hurt a lot. I came down really hard on my tailbone," I said, my shoulders shaking through my tears.

"Let's move to the side and take a break. Do you think you can keep going?"

"I'm not sure what other choice I have. I'll be fine. Let's just go."

"Are you sure," he said. "I think you should rest a little longer. It's still a long way down."

"Bob, I'm fine. Let's go." I said a bit too forcefully. Not only was I physically hurt, but I was embarrassed as well.

"Well, you lead the way so that you can set the pace. Go as slowly as you need to."

Thankfully, both my position in the front of the group and my sunglasses hid the tears that wouldn't stop streaming down my face for a good five minutes. Not only was I embarrassed for falling in the first place, but I felt stupid for crying.

I guess there was a little bit of silver lining in the situation, though. My tailbone hurt so bad that it made me forget about how tired my leg was. I felt pain with every single step. When we finally got to the bottom, I was relieved to say the least. However, when I sat down in the passenger seat of Christie's car, all that relief was instantly obliterated. It brought tears to my eyes all over again just to put direct pressure on my tailbone. I braced myself by clutching the door handle with my right hand and the center console with my left. I lifted my butt a little to ease the pain.

"Well, this flight tomorrow is going to be interesting," I said with a half-smile.

"Good thing it's only a couple hours," Bob said sympathetically. "I could get you one of those doughnut things to sit on," he joked.

"Not funny," I said, even though it kind of was.

It took two weeks before I could sit comfortably. But, even through all the pain, I was still glad that I did it. This might sound corny, but when I have a challenging task ahead of me, I think of Camelback. There aren't too many things that are as physically taxing as climbing a mountain. In comparison to that, obstacles don't seem nearly as daunting.

- - -

Bob teaching at a private school has its perks. Every other summer he puts together a trip to his chosen location(s) during the summer through EF Tours. The company prides itself on educational tours where students can learn more about the world and have great, hands on experiences. So far, we've gotten to go to France, England, Germany, Austria, Belgium, Hawaii, New Zealand, and Australia as chaperones. We cannot wait to take our kids with us when they get old enough so we can teach them about other cultures and languages. But for now, we typically take anywhere between 60-70 of his high school students with us on the trips.

Two summers ago, our first stop was to Cairns, Australia, which I ignorantly didn't know was pronounced like "cans" until I got there. The first thing on our itinerary was to go snorkeling in the Great Barrier Reef. As soon as I saw that, I grew tense. Like I mentioned before, water and I don't really get along. I wasn't worried about my swimming capability but wondered how in the world I was going to snorkel without two fins.

"Won't I just go in a circle?" I asked Bob.

161

"How would I know?" he laughed. "In case you missed it, I *have* two feet. I'm sure we can figure it out though. You're not coming all the way here and sitting this one out."

"Oh, I want to. I just don't know if I *can*."

"Let's just get out there and then ask someone that's in charge, ok?"

Our group of 27 people boarded the boat around 8:00 a.m. along with hundreds of other people. It was raining and about fifty degrees, which is abnormally cold for their Winter season. All of us were freezing in our sweatshirt and long pants, wondering how in the world they were going to get us into the water when we were already that cold.

About twenty minutes after the boat left port, a few people started getting sick. The workers handed them puke bags. We didn't think anything of it. Our tour guide had suggested that we all take Dramamine in order to avoid getting seasick, and we heeded her advice. We didn't want a chance of a lifetime to be ruined by feeling ill. Of course, after we mocked the people who were throwing up, some of the students in our group started feeling sick.

"Didn't you take your medicine like I told you?" Bob asked them.

"Yes, but it's not working."

Soon after, one of our other chaperones, Rob, grabbed a bag from the worker and put the entire contents of his breakfast inside. Rob is 6'3" and over 300 pounds, so it was a lot of breakfast.

Our tour guide, Anya, was making her way around checking on everyone. "Go outside. You must go outside," she said in her German accent. "Just look at the horizon. You will feel much better."

"I don't feel so hot," Bob said.

"Oh no. Not you too. Alright, come on. Let's go outside."

As soon as we did, we instantly felt better. We were soaking wet from the rain and were bitterly cold, but it was much better than puking our guts out.

When we arrived at our destination to go snorkeling, the captain announced over the PA, "There will be a lunch buffet in about fifteen minutes."

"Oh my gosh. I don't even want to *think* about food," Bob said.

"Ugh, me either," said Rob. "You wanna just jump right in the water?" he asked Bob.

"I'm not eating, that's for sure. Yeah, let's do it."

Right at that minute, a huge storm blew in. The wind and rain picked up, and everyone went inside to eat. Standing on the dock, we were all fiercely shivering so badly that our teeth were chattering.

"I'm doing it," Rob said as he bravely took the plunge. "The water is actually warmer than out there. Get in," he told Bob.

Following suit, Bob jumped in too.

"How is it," I yelled to him?

"It's awesome! The water *is* warmer. You should come in."

Still unsure about the whole snorkeling thing, I decided to go in and eat in the warmth with two of our other female chaperones. We had some of the most amazing food that we'd ever had. I tried so many new things, dragon fruit probably being my favorite.

After lunch was over, one of the chaperones that I ate with, Kassidy, said that she wanted to go into the water with her husband Rob. I went out onto the dock with her as she got suited up with the correct size flippers and mask. She turned to me and said, "Are you getting in?"

"Yeah, I think I'm going to try. Once you get in, will you ask Bob to come back here and help me get in?"

I took my leg off and handed it over to one of our friends, Amy. She wrapped it in a towel and took it to a safe place where it wouldn't get wet. Then, I put a flipper on my left foot, grabbed a mask, and sat down on the metal platform that served as an entrance to the water. I didn't wait long before Bob swam up.

"Ready?" he asked.

"I think so," I said, grabbed his hand. The metal had slats in it, which hurt the end of my stump as I tried to walk across it

Bob saw me grimace. "Why don't you just slide on your butt instead of trying to walk?"

"That's a good idea," I said, doing as he suggested. Once I got to the end of the platform, I pushed off it with my left leg and started swimming.

"Put your face in the water," Bob said.

"I don't want to touch the fish!" I said, surprised at how afraid I was. I didn't grow up swimming in ponds like Bob did. I'm a suburban girl through and through. To me, swimming meant a pool with no animals!

I got the courage to put my face in, but as soon as I did, I felt a tap on my shoulder. I looked up and saw Bob pointing down into the water in the opposite direction that I was facing. There, about a foot away from me, was a gigantic fish. I popped up so quickly with my eyes wide open in fear.

"What the heck is that thing?" I asked him.

He started dying laughing. "That's a grouper. It's the biggest one I've ever seen." It was probably the length of him at around 6' 2". "I saw it as soon as I jumped in. I didn't want to tell you because I knew you wouldn't get in if you knew."

"Well, you're probably right about that."

The longer I stayed in the ocean, the more comfortable I felt. The Great Barrier Reef was hands down the most amazing thing that I have ever seen. The corral was enormous and so vibrantly colored. I couldn't believe the sheer number of fish that surrounded me and was pleased at the fact that they seemed more afraid of me than I was of them. Every time that I got close, they would dart away. But, all of a sudden, hundreds of fish started swarming me. I could feel them touching me on every square inch of my body. I frantically popped my head out of the water again to see if I could figure out what had changed to make them act that way. The second I did, I saw Bob hysterically laughing...again.

"What the heck was that?" I yelled.

"The lifeguard threw fish food right on top of you."

"Are you serious?! Why would he do that?"

"I don't know. Maybe he sensed your fear," Bob said, still laughing.

"This is NOT funny," I said

"Maybe just a little bit?"

I rolled my eyes at him, which he must be pretty used to by now. I mentioned before that I fell in love with Bob because he always challenged me to be a better person. This situation was no different. Because I tend to take life a bit too seriously, he is constantly trying to get me to loosen up and have more fun. After the initial shock of the fish incident had worn off, and after Bob's prodding, I eventually did see the humor in it.

About thirty minutes later, our group was scheduled to go on an excursion with a marine biologist.

"Are you up for this?" Bob asked me.

"Yeah, I think so. I just don't want to hold anyone up."

"I doubt anyone would care. It'll give us more time to look at things. But we'll be gone for thirty minutes. You have that in you?"

"I actually can't believe how easy it's been so far. The salt water makes us really buoyant, so I don't feel tired at all."

I saw that the marine biologist held a yellow, circular flotation device, which eased my mind even more. He instructed us to grab on if we needed a break and he would pull us along.

Our group consisted of the marine biologist and six chaperones. We ventured away from the boat and all the other people in order to see more ocean life and more unique coral. It was crazy how easy it was to tell the differences in water depth based on the temperature. Overall, the water was colder than I would have liked. Most of the natives wear a wetsuit in the winter, but we were too naive and cheap.

Bob and Rob, the more adventurous of the group, were out in front of everyone, exploring on their own. I, on the other hand, was more timid and stayed close to the marine biologist and his life ring. About halfway through our tour, we came to a spot where the coral was very close to the surface.

"Whatever you do, don't touch the coral," said the marine biologist. "There are also a ton of sea turtles in this area, but make sure you don't touch them either. They're protected."

I'm sure we all tried our hardest not to touch the coral, but it was almost impossible. There just simply wasn't enough room between our bodies and the reef. I hit it a couple of times with my left foot, but it wasn't painful because my flipper acted as a shield. But, my stump didn't have any protection, so my shin got scraped up pretty badly. Thankfully, it only hurt right when I did it, but the pain dissipated quickly... until I put my prosthesis on when we got back to the boat. The hard plastic rubbing against the sore was very painful, but also unavoidable. I had to wear it to walk, so I just dealt with it.

Oddly enough, we accidentally broke the marine biologist's second rule as well. He was right. There were quite a few sea turtles floating around. Bob was right in front of me at the time, and out of nowhere, one came swimming right at him. I could tell that he tried to dodge it, but unable to react quickly enough, bumped right into it. The turtles were so beautiful. I had never seen one up close before, and the water was so clear that I could make out every little detail. Rule broken or not, it was one of the highlights of not only the entire trip, but my life. The Great Barrier Reef is so vast and beautiful. Nothing that I could write would ever do it justice.

There was only one thing on the return trip to the boat that took my mind off the beauty. Because my left leg was doing the work of two, I got a severe cramp in my calf. I tried to stretch, but it was hard to do in the middle of the ocean. I grabbed my leg with both hands and pulled my toes toward me. My muscles were so fatigued that I didn't know if I could keep going. Thankfully, we were within five minutes of the boat, so I grabbed onto the marine biologist's ring and let him pull me in the rest of the way.

When we got back, my group wanted to stay in the water, but I knew that wasn't an option for me. Amy was tired from the swim too, so she and I decided to get out and go on a glass bottom boat tour. Bob helped me get out of the water, and Amy went to fetch my prosthesis. Even though I was bummed that I had to cut my snorkeling adventure short, it actually worked out in my favor. Amy and I were able to see a shark, albeit a small one, through the glass on the bottom of the boat. After seeing that, going back into the water was not an option and just reaffirmed my no swimming with animals policy.

166

Just like my other two ventures, snorkeling in the Great Barrier Reef was one of my proudest moments. It wasn't as challenging as climbing a mountain, and it didn't take as much preparation as running a 5K, but it got me out of my comfort zone, helped me tackle a life-long fear, and let me see the amazing things that I can experience if I let my guard down enough to forget about my reservations.

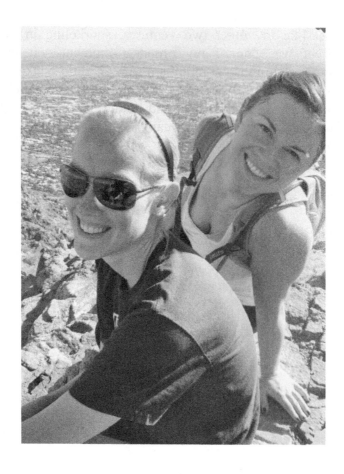

Christie and I at the top of Camelback Mountain in Phoenix, Arizona.

Chapter 15

Another New Prosthesis

A good fitting prosthesis becomes like that worn, threadbare shirt that you've had for nearly a decade. The shirt might have holes in it, and you probably never venture out in public with it anymore, but you can't bear the thought of throwing it away. My current prosthesis is exactly that. At five-years-old, it's finally starting to show its age. The skin is ripping, and the locking mechanism has completely dislodged from the bottom of the socket. My old prosthetist, Travis, tried to reattach it with silicone about a year ago, but it only lasted a few days before it worked itself free again. With that being said, I never made a maintenance appointment with Optimus Prosthetics to get it fixed. I knew that they would tell me I needed a new leg, and I just wasn't ready to give up my Linus blanket.

Most people would think I'm crazy for waiting a year to get my prosthesis fixed, but the malfunctioning lock wasn't as big of an issue as what it seems. The only time the lock dislodged is when I got down into a kneeling position. Otherwise, it fit like a glove, broken-in and comfortable. I probably would have waited even longer if Optimus' receptionist, Andrea, hadn't called me to touch base because it had been so long since I'd been in their office.

Upon arriving at the office, I discovered that Travis was no longer employed there, having moved to Columbus, Ohio. Just like amputees often become emotionally attached to their prostheses, we tend to have the same feeling about our prosthetists. Travis and I had worked together for five years, so he was aware of what I wanted out of a prosthesis and understood my hesitancy to change. For example, he knew that I preferred him to cast me in the "old school" way that Wayne did all those years ago rather than 3-D scanning. Casting had always given me better results. I got spoiled having Wayne as my prosthetist at The Shriners Medical Center for nearly my entire childhood. Although it's expected that there is turnover in every job, I wished that I could keep being Travis' patient for as long as I was Wayne's.

Seeing as how that was obviously not an option, I was told that Derick Schmidt was going to be my new prosthetist. Within the first minute of our consultation, my fear became reality; Derick told me that my prosthesis was irreparable and that I would need to be fitted for a new one. We started discussing new technology, my needs, activity level, and hopes for my device. He showed me a picture on Ossur's website of the LP Align foot, which was the newest foot on the market and just released to the public three months prior. Immediately, I started getting excited when I saw that I could potentially wear dress shoes with even higher heels than before and have a more durable foot.

"That is perfect," I told Derick. "It's exactly what I want."

He paused for a second to study my prosthesis. "Hold on. Don't get too excited yet. The LP Align is a lot taller than your current foot."

"And I assume that's a problem?"

"Well, your stump is so long that I don't think there's going to be enough room at the bottom of your socket to put the pin."

"So, what do we do?" I asked. "Is there another option?"

"We could switch to suction. You wouldn't need a pin since the suction apparatus is an extra, partial-liner that you pull on over top of your normal liner. Have you ever had a prosthesis held on by suction before?"

"Ugh, don't remind me. I *hate* suction! I had it in middle school, and it fell off a lot. I've had a locking liner ever since, and I've been very satisfied with it overall. Are you sure we can't stick with the lock and pin method?"

"Well, suction has really changed a lot since then. This wouldn't be partial-suction like you had before. It would have a one-way valve to ensure no air gets in to break the seal. We could give it a try."

"I dunno. I'm still a little leery about it. What if I get it and end up hating it?"

"That's why we do test sockets."

I decided to give it a try, knowing that I wouldn't know if a better option existed if I wasn't open to change. Before leaving the office that day, Derick also informed me that insurance companies have restricted the process of getting a prosthesis, and that I would now have to get a prescription from a doctor.

"Let me get this right—doctors now have to tell amputees that we need a prosthesis? We're amputees. Of *course* we need a prosthesis."

"I guess too many amputees were trying to get a device every year. It got so expensive that they had to start restricting it. They're trying to determine if it's a need versus a want."

"I guess that makes sense," I replied.

We went ahead and scheduled a tele-med appointment two weeks from then with a doctor that Derick recommended. It kept me from having to drive all over creation because I could tele-med at Optimus and have my fitting appointment directly after. Talk about convenience!

When I returned to Optimus a couple weeks later, I was ushered back to one of the patient rooms. Derick came in with his computer so that we could video chat with the doctor. After I caught the doctor up to speed about my medical history, he asked, "Can you show me where your prosthesis is broken?"

I held my leg up for him to see, but it was difficult for him to decipher since he wasn't there in person.

"No abrasions on your skin?" he asked.

"No, not right now."

"Can I please see you walk?"

Derick grabbed his computer so that he could follow me with the camera as I moved throughout the room.

"Wow, very fluid. What types of activities do you do that would warrant a certain device?"

"Well, I roller blade, ride my bike, go on walks, do workout videos, mow the grass... things like that."

He paused for a while, seeming to think of how to phrase his next response. "If I'm being completely honest, I think you're going to have a tough time getting your insurance company to approve a new device."

"Really? Why is that?" I asked.

"Because you're too healthy."

"Too healthy?" I started to get a little defensive. "Why would that matter? Do you think they would miss the part when we tell them that my prosthesis is *broken*?" I asked, probably a little too harshly.

"I'm just saying that I've seen people get denied that weren't nearly as active and healthy as you. If someone has diabetes or is significantly overweight, they seem to always have their device approved."

I appreciated his honesty, but from that point forward, I wasn't too optimistic. I waited for Derick to leave the room to get his casting supplies before getting my phone out of my purse to call Bob.

"What do you mean they might not cover it?" Bob asked.

"I guess the insurance companies have really started to reign things in, and apparently I'm 'too healthy.'"

"That makes no sense," he said, dumbfounded. "Worst case scenario—how much would we have to pay?"

"The leg costs $11,000."

"Well, it is what it is. Obviously, we'll pray that insurance *does* cover it, but if they don't, you need a new leg, Kendra. We'll just have to pay it."

"I know. We have the money, but you know me… I'm cheap, and I didn't foresee us having to use our savings on this."

"Well, that's why we have a savings. Let's try not to worry about it until we know for sure that they won't pay for it."

Derick came back into the room with his hands full of supplies. I could tell he was totally in his element. "Have you ever done a three-part casting?" he asked, smiling.

"Nope. Never even heard of it," I told him. "What is it?"

"In addition to casting you with your leg completely straight, I will also do one with your knee bent. That gives the prosthesis a more versatile design because it accounts for the many positions that you're in throughout the day."

"I like the sound of that. I bet that will give me a better fit instead of it always digging into me every time I bend my leg. What's that, though?" I asked as I pointed to the machine on the ground.

"Oh, that's a vacuum," Derick said.

"Hmm, it sure doesn't look like the Dyson vacuum that I'm used to," I laughed. "And I assume it's not going to sweep the floor either."

"Yeah, not so much. It will help get all the air bubbles out of the cast so that it's a perfect fit." He plugged the cord into the outlet, and it came to life, emitting a constant, low grumbling noise. While the vacuum was warming up, Derick instructed me to put on my liner. He then placed a thin, plastic bag over it to keep it from getting dirty. Derick reached down and grabbed the same type of white, cylindrical roll that my first prosthetist used over thirty years ago.

"You don't like 3D scanning either?" I asked.

"Not really. I need to feel the limb with my hands. I can make minor adjustments to account for problem areas that the scanner doesn't pick up on. I truly believe in three-part casting." A vision of an artist around a pottery wheel came to my mind, molding the clay in his hands with precision and grace.

Derick dipped the roll into the water and unraveled it on the lower portion of my liner. He smoothed it out with his hands and contoured it around my tibia bone, which as I mentioned earlier, tends to give me problems. The contouring left some extra space so that my bone wouldn't rub directly against the hard socket.

"Alright, we're ready for the vacuum," Derick said. He attached the end of the vacuum to a valve in the bag. As soon as he did that, I could feel the plastic shrink against my liner as the excess air was removed. When everything was to Derick's liking, he turned off the vacuum and said, "I'm going to add more layers above that now so that I can get your knee. Go ahead and completely extend your leg."

I did as I was told while he continued to wrap me like a mummy.

"Before it dries and becomes less malleable, I'm going to do the third part. Bend your knee, and I'll start to smooth it out."

"Can you make sure to leave a little space on the sides of my knee? That's another problem area."

"Sure. I'll press out on those areas as the vacuum is running to give you more room." Derick turned the machine back on and repeated the same process as before. "Ok, now if everything worked right, the whole cast should just slide off when I pull it." He gave the now hardened cast a little tug, and off it came.

"Isn't that cool!" I said in awe.

Derick gave me a little smile. I could tell he was pleased with the product that he created. He wrote my name on the cast with a black sharpie marker and started the clean up process.

"Where do we go from here, Derick?" I asked.

"It'll take me about a week to make this into a test socket. I'll have Andrea call you to set up an appointment."

I left the office that day feeling hopeful. The three-part casting was such a neat concept that I thought it *had* to produce a more comfortable socket.

When I returned to Optimus Prosthetics a week later to pick up the test socket, I didn't even get halfway through the main door before Andrea exclaimed, "Insurance approved your leg!" Her perfect, blonde curls bounced when she said it. I could tell she'd been staring at the door, excitedly anticipating my arrival. She couldn't wait to give me the good news. Andrea is bubbly and outgoing by nature, but her excitement was ramped up another notch during that moment. A potential problem that didn't directly involve her shouldn't have mattered, but it did. It's reasons like this that I stay with Optimus.

"They did?" I said, my voice filled with relief.

"We literally just got the approval thirty minutes ago," Andrea said.

"Perfect timing! It's crazy how one phone call can instantly resolve an $11,000 problem," I joked.

"No kidding! To add to the good news, I have something for you, too. Take a look at this list and pick a shirt design that you like," Andrea said as she handed me a laminated sheet of paper. "We're giving them away for free."

174

The choices were as follows: "Some Assembly Required" with a picture of stick figures missing various limbs, "I'm only in it for the parking" above a handicapped symbol, "The only disability in life is a bad attitude," and an acrostic poem spelling AMPUTEE going vertically down the shirt that read:

Always
Motivates
Perseveres
Under
Tough
Encounters
Everyday

I looked at the list for quite some time, finding it difficult to make up my mind.

"Man, this is tough. I like them all. I guess I'll take the 'Some Assembly Required' one. It's hilarious!"

"I'm glad you think so," Andrea said. "I always get a little anxious before handing the list to people. I never know how they're going to react."

"Oh, really? Why's that?"

"Well, some people just aren't ready. They can't see the humor in it yet."

"That's understandable. I can't even imagine. I say this all the time, but I'm fortunate that I lost my leg so early in life."

"Yeah, but you have such a good attitude about it. I wish more people could have that mentality, but I do understand that it takes time," Andrea said.

"Oh yeah. It's an ongoing battle. I've had 32 years to develop this attitude. Some of the people that come here have only had a few years or even months."

After I got my shirt, Derick came down the hallway holding a clear, test socket.

"I'm guessing that's mine," I said to him.

"Sure is. Come on in and we'll see how it fits."

I sat down in a chair and started removing my prosthesis. I carefully rolled on the new, thicker liner. Upon doing so, I could feel a pocket of air form at the bottom. I put one hand on top of the liner and one on bottom and squeezed as hard as I could while moving upward toward my knee. As I did, the air bubble came out the top of the liner.

"This liner sure does trap a lot of air," I said.

"That's probably because your stump goes from being thick to skinny really quickly here at the bottom. I'm guessing, because of the thickness, the liner isn't molding to your leg as well," Derick explained.

"Is there any way to fix that?"

"Not unless you want to switch to a custom liner."

"And I'm guessing custom means expensive?"

"Pretty much," Derrick said.

"Well, let's try to make this work. Maybe it will be better when I put it all on." I slipped the other partial liner on top of the liner I was already wearing. It contained three tiny, circular rings that helped to create the seal. When everything was in place, I stood up and balanced on my left leg while I waited for Derick to put my socket in front of me. I stepped down into it and felt the air release out of the one-way valve.

"Can I walk on it?" I asked Derick.

"Yeah, but don't do anything crazy on it yet. Test sockets aren't very durable." I was all too aware of that. When I was younger, I tried on my first ever test socket. Wayne failed to warn me that it wasn't yet the robust, finished product that I was used to. Within seconds of putting it on, I jumped on it and instantly fell to the ground. The test socket had a clean, circular crack around the middle. I remember picking up the two pieces and just staring at Wayne, still too shocked to form words. All his work was ruined in the matter of seconds.

Learning my lesson from years prior, I gingerly set off to take my first step on my new trial leg. As I stepped down, I slightly lost my balance. "Whoa. That's crazy!" I exclaimed.

"What is?" Derick asked.

"The ankle moves so much. I wasn't ready for it. It's like I'm actually walking heel to toe. I've never felt anything like this in my life. It's so realistic, almost like how I walk with my left leg."

"That's great! Do you want to go in between the metal bars so that you can hold on until you get used to it? Derick asked.

"Nah, I'm good. I do still feel some air though. I can't tell if it's still in the liner or if it's in the socket itself."

"It might be because the material that we use for the test socket is a little bit more flexible. Air could be finding a way in somehow. But, when we finish it out and use the harder, laminated plastic, it shouldn't be a problem," Derick explained.

I continued to walk around the room, pausing every once in a while for Derrick to make some minor modifications.

"I feel like I'm walking on the outside of my foot too much. Can you adjust that so that I hit more in the middle?"

"That's crazy that you can feel that. It's obvious that you've had a prosthesis for a long time. People who are new to this process don't know any different. You know what to look for and when things seem off."

"It is a gift and a curse," I said. "I bet it's harder to work with patients like me. We're a lot more high-maintenance, huh?"

"I wouldn't say it like that exactly..." Derick laughed.

"Yeah, that's because you're being nice."

I don't think I've ever been faulted for being high-maintenance in any other facet of my life. In fact, I'm quite the opposite. However, I unfortunately gave congenital amputees a bad rap again. Not only did I ask him to make me a different test socket, I had him create a *third*!

The first test socket was putting a lot of pressure on the bottom of my stump and caused it to become red and swollen. Derick modified the mold to add more space at the bottom to combat the issue. Although the change helped a little, it didn't completely rectify the problem. In fact, I couldn't even bare to wear the socket for more than a couple of hours at a time.

After hearing that the new test socket still wasn't up to my standards, Derick called me to try to figure out a different solution.

"Hey, I think I have something that might help the pain you're having. I know you've come into the office a lot lately, and it's a bit of a drive. I go past your exit every day on my way home. Do you want to meet somewhere so that I can save you a trip?"

"Oh my gosh. That would be awesome. There's a new Chipotle right off the Monroe exit. Would that work?"

I'll admit that a restaurant's parking lot is an odd place for a leg exchange, but meeting there saved me an hour and a half drive on multiple occasions. On that specific day, Derick brought me a silicone disc that he wanted me to insert into the bottom of the socket.

"Try this out. It will give you extra padding and hopefully take some of the pressure off the end of your leg."

This small change ended up being the exact solution that I needed. However, now that I was able to wear the socket for the entire day, I was able to pick up on another problem area. There was a spot right under my knee that kept digging into the bone.

After three consecutive days of exclusively wearing the test socket, I called it quits.

"I cannot wear this thing one second longer," I told Bob as I took it off to show him how red and inflamed my stump had become.

"Yeah, that doesn't look good. I would stop wearing it too. I don't think the goal is to suffer through it and be miserable. You're just trying to see if the test socket fits properly. You don't really need any more time to figure out that it's not."

"You're right, but I'm so frustrated. I don't know if we'll ever get this socket right."

"Has it ever been this difficult before?" Bob asked.

"No. I've always just had one test socket. I don't know why we're having such a hard time with this one."

The next day I called and told Derick the bad news. He had me drive down to the office so he could attempt to fix the problem area. I pointed to the spot where it was hurting, and he used a marker to draw a line so he would know what area needed work. Derick went to the lab, located in the back of Optimus Prosthetics, to make his modifications while I remained in the patient room.

While in the lab, he heated up the plastic, reached his hand down into the socket, and pushed out in order to make more room. When he returned, I tried on the socket to see if the problem was resolved.

"Well, I see a problem already," Derick said.

"You do?"

"Yeah, you're losing a little bit of suction. Do you see how only two of the three rings are being pressed down to create the seal now?"

"Oh yeah. That's not good."

"Why don't you sit down, and I will try to pull the socket off of you to see how much the suction has been compromised."

"Ok…" I said, laughing at how unscientific this test was going to be.

Derick grabbed my foot and started to pull with as much fervor as he could muster. The socket didn't budge at first, but he did manage to scoot the chair that I was on halfway across the room. It wasn't until the very end of the pulling process that the socket eventually came off.

"Well, I think we're good to go. If it was that difficult to get off, I don't think it's going anywhere," Derick said.

After the adjustments were made, I tried the socket for another three days. The changes improved my comfort level, but only slightly. Because Derick couldn't push that exact location out any more without further compromising the suction, it was decided that a third test socket had to be made.

Maybe there is some validity behind the cliché expression "third time's a charm" because it sure held true for me. Since the test socket finally fit to my liking, we decided to move forward in the process. Three weeks later, I returned to Optimus Prosthetics to retrieve my finished product.

However, when Derick came into the room holding only a somewhat finished prosthesis, I was caught off-guard.

"Now, I know you were expecting this to have the foam and skin on it, but I thought we should leave it like this for a while so we can do minor tweaks. We can't adjust the angle of the foot or the height of the leg if the skin is on," he explained.

"Oh, that makes sense," I said. "That's probably a good idea." After the surprise of not seeing it finished wore off, I took a good, long look at the leg. I started to feel a bit unsettled by what I saw. "Derick, are you going to be able to hide the valve once the foam and skin are put on? It sticks out a lot. I don't want a big bulge on the side of my leg."

"I see what you're saying. I'll obviously be able to hide it some, but I don't think we'll be able to mask it entirely." I let out a big sigh, not really caring if Derick picked up on my disappointment. "It's hard with your leg because it's so skinny," he told me. "For other people, we can hide it better, but there's just no place to do it for you."

Without knowing what the finished product would look like, I began to think of the worst. I know it seems vain, but I couldn't have a leg that I wear all day every day have a giant goose egg protruding from the side. I had made so much progress with the appearance of my prothesis in the last decade. For me to take such a big step backward was deflating to say the least.

"I promise I'll do my best," Derick reassured me. "Let's take measurements of your left leg so that I can try to make it as close of a match as possible, ok?" He proceeded to measure my calf and ankle circumference and took pictures of the front and side profile of my left leg.

Knowing that he was going through great lengths to make my legs match to the best of his ability gave me the reassurance I was looking for. Derick quickly adjusted the foot alignment and instructed me to come back in a few weeks for him to finish it the rest of the way.

Before leaving, I stopped at the front desk to pay the remaining portion of the bill that insurance didn't cover. Since my deductible and out of pocket expenses for the year were almost met, I was only responsible for $1,200. When compared to the $11,000 that I could have paid, it was a bargain.

It didn't take long to notice that the socket was the best fitting of all the prostheses that I've ever owned. There was not one single place on my stump that I considered even mildly uncomfortable.

With the socket fitting so well, you would assume that I was quick to get my prosthesis completed. However, after a week of wearing it, I started to notice another problem. This one was even more severe. When I would walk at a fast pace, my prosthesis would lose suction in between steps. Thankfully, my leg would only partially come off. By the time I put my full weight on it, it would regain its seal.

I scheduled yet another appointment with Derick to brainstorm a different solution. The night before the appointment, I went to my daughter's school for a family movie night. We grabbed a bag of popcorn when we entered, said hi to some of her friends, and then walked up the bleachers until we found a place to sit. At the conclusion of the movie, families started filing out of the gym. The stairs on the bleachers were crowded, so I impatiently decided to get down faster by stepping on the seat tops. However, it was a big drop from one row to the next. As I was stepping down, my prosthesis completely came off. It slid down until I heard it hit the bleachers. I was sure I was going to fall on my face. Thankfully, a man close by was paying attention and came to my rescue. He grabbed my right arm and steadied me, saving me from embarrassment and possible injury.

I shared the story with Derick the next day. "Well, we can't have that happening," he said.

"I am so sorry. I'm not trying to be difficult, but I can't have a leg that falls off."

Since then, he has ordered me three other types of suction liners to see if any of them would resolve the problem. However, Derick and I worked out a backup plan in case none of them do. We would have to start all over and go back to a locking liner, but he thinks I could keep the foot that I like. I know that Optimus Prosthetics will do whatever it takes to provide me with a prosthesis that works, even if that means eating some of the cost for the remake.

Although this process has been long and frustrating, I don't doubt Derick's competence or Optimus Prosthetic's capability one bit. This is a custom, personalized limb that we're talking about, not a mass-produced Nike shoe that I can get right off the shelf. It takes time, patience, a lot of adjustment, and maybe even a little luck. The fitting process is far from over for this particular prosthesis, but I'm confident that I will eventually have a leg that is not only functional, but beautiful as well. Who knows, maybe it will eventually become like that tattered old t-shirt that I just can't seem to part with.

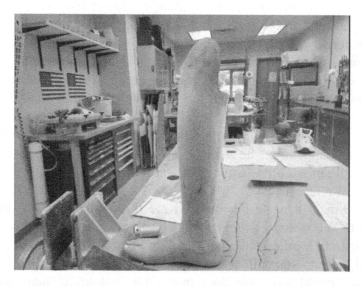

This is my new leg that is in the fabrication stage. My prosthetist just finished molding the foam to match the shape of my left leg in order to give it a more realistic look. The next step is to put the skin on it.

Chapter 16

The Joys of Aging

I won't be dramatic and say that 34 years old is *old*. But, being an amputee has definitely gotten harder as I've aged. For starters, sores on my leg don't heal as quickly. In high school and college, if I overdid it in the gym the night before and caused myself to get some kind of skin abrasion, it would be gone in a day or two if I made a point to leave my prosthesis off a little more than normal. But even in my late twenties, I could tell I was having to nurse it more carefully.

I mentioned before that I can only recall a handful of times that I have had to use crutches. Two of those days came when I was teaching at Middletown. I had a very strenuous workout one evening, and my stump was sweating so badly that my liner kept sliding down. I went to the bathroom two or three times at the gym to sop up the sweat with my towel, but I couldn't keep up with it. I didn't notice it at the time, but when I got home, I could tell that the friction caused a spot on my knee to be rubbed raw. Of course, my socket pressed right against that spot each time that I took a step.

I tried to power through it the next day at work, but the more I walked, the worse it became. For the average person, a little sore on his/her leg the size of a quarter wouldn't be a big deal, but for me, it was the type of pain that required me to battle against my mind to even stand up and put pressure on my leg. A lot of people have told me that I have amazing will power and strong mental fortitude. I'm sure God has something to do with that, but it wasn't developed overnight. It was moments like this that developed that characteristic. The internal battles that I had against the voices that told me to stop, sit down, and give up helped me to become this way.

After coming home almost in tears, I decided that the only way that I could get through the next day was to use my crutches. My students were taken aback; they had never seen me use them before.

"Herber, what's wrong? Did you sprain your ankle or something?" a student asked.

"Oh no, I'm just having a bad leg day," I explained.

"What does that mean?"

"I have a sore on my stump, and if I don't let it rest, it'll keep getting worse."

"Then why don't you have it off?" my student asked.

"Well, I had to drive here, but it's also nice to know that if I have to catch my balance or something, I can."

"You don't need it on to teach. Why don't you just take it off? You can sit in your rolly chair and scoot around," she suggested.

"Yeah, and we can help pass out the papers. We got you, Herber," another student chimed in.

I couldn't believe they were so empathetic. Middletown High School has a bad reputation and doesn't do well on the state report card, but I have never had a group of students that made me feel the way those kids did that day. In my experience, Middletown students were some of the most caring and loyal kids I've ever taught.

After I came back from lunch, I saw a piece of paper on my desk that said, "open me" on the front. On the inside there was a hand drawn picture of a llama that had a prosthetic leg. At the top it said, "Get well soon, you llama loving lady." Not only did this student know my strange obsession with llamas, but she apparently had also been listening to my lesson on alliteration.

However, recovery time isn't the only issue that has reared its ugly head. As of late, I've also had to deal with atrophy. It's not like I just woke up one day and realized that my stump had gotten skinnier. It took years for me to notice. The first indication was when my tibia bone started to give me problems. The little muscle that I did have in my leg started to shrink and the skin on top of my tibia was very thin, providing little cushion.

When I was younger, I remember by grandpa telling me to do exercises every day to ensure that this exact problem didn't happen. But, like most young people, I thought I knew it all and didn't heed his advice. I'm kicking myself for that now because my prosthetist, Derick, recently told me that once the muscle is gone, it's

184

almost impossible for amputees to gain it back or reverse the effects of atrophy. There is simply no way to be active enough to combat the rate of muscle deterioration that is already occurring. Right now, the only thing that I can do is make sure that I don't lose any more.

Both Derick and I have made some changes to fix the issue. I, for one, have started doing stump exercises every morning before I put on my prosthesis. I wiggle it forward twenty times and backwards twenty times. When I first started these exercises about three months ago, I couldn't even do ten consecutively. Now, the twenty seem effortless, and I am hoping to increase that number so that I can rebuild those muscles. I know Derick said that I can't reverse the effects of atrophy, but if I can already tell that I'm stronger, then maybe it *is* possible...

One of the ways that Derick has tried to combat my pain from atrophy is by giving me a thicker liner. Instead of a 3mm one, I now use a 6mm. That might not seem like a big difference, but doubling the padding means that my bone isn't rubbing against the hard, laminate socket. It has increased my comfort substantially.

However, my stump isn't the only part of me that has started to atrophy; my right thigh has as well. It might not be evident to other people at this point, but to me, it's very apparent. When I'm wearing pants, the fabric is tight against my left thigh and loose on my right. I can pull the fabric away from my skin about an inch.

Similarly, when I go on long bike rides, I wear biking shorts that have padding in them. The end of the shorts has elastic to ensure they don't ride up. Because I have a small waist, I find it difficult to buy shorts that fit both my skinny midsection and muscular legs. I found a pair of shorts that fit the best, but they weren't perfect by any means. The right leg fit fine since it is thinner, but I had to cut a two-inch slit in the elastic on my left leg because it was cutting off my circulation.

I try my hardest not to compensate for my lack of a foot. If I don't concentrate on using my right leg during exercise, my body subconsciously does whatever is easiest. I am constantly fighting against my brain's natural tendencies so that I can strengthen the muscles in my right leg. Simple things like going up and down stairs are tasks that I have to be more cognizant of. I tend to always step down with my left leg first and keep my right leg completely straight as it follows behind. It almost looks as if I am galloping down the stairs. When I do squats, I favor my left leg by bearing most of my weight on it rather than sharing the burden. While riding a bike, I have to make sure that I am pushing equally as hard with my right leg as I am with my left. If not, I tend to push extra hard with my good leg so that when the pedal comes back around to my bad side, it's easier because I've already done most of the work. It is my hope that since I have the fight in me to still try to combat these issues, I can at least prolong the negative effects of atrophy.

- - -

As I've gotten older, I have developed mild arthritis in my knee. It is already so much smaller and underdeveloped than my other one, so it makes sense that my knee joint is starting to become inflamed. I only notice the arthritic pain after I do a high impact workout. When doing high knees, box jumps, or ski jumps during Insanity or other Beach Body workouts, I notice the dull ache in my knee the day after. Running is the biggest culprit. I feel pain almost immediately if I so much as even try to do interval training. My smaller than normal knee is forced to absorb all the impact, and it simply cannot handle it.

I've had to alter my workouts to make sure I'm not in too much pain. I never do two days in a row of high impact training. In fact, the last year or so I have almost given it up entirely. The competitor in me really misses the challenge. It's yet another instance where I'm frustrated by my limitations, defenseless against the changes that my body is going through. Everything in me wants to power through and do it anyway, but I know the consequences of that all too well.

Instead, I've had to modify the movements to a lower impact version of the same exercise. Recently, I purchased a Kinetic Road Machine Bike Trainer that I put in my basement for the winter so that I could get my cardio in despite the cold weather. The bike trainer stabilizes my back tire and provides resistance so that I can still get a good workout. Riding a bike strengthens my knee and counteracts the effects of arthritis.

On my bad leg days when it hurts to even wear my prosthesis, I still find ways to workout. I get on YouTube and search for 30-minute floor exercises. My favorite one is "30 Minute No Impact Total Body Floor Barre For Healing, Strength, and Fitness." I take off my prosthesis and spend 30 minutes strengthening my whole body while never once getting off the floor. I have to admit that there aren't too many workouts like this. It's been my dream for a few years now to make my own workout video. I would film the whole thing without my prosthesis on. I'm sure there are other amputees out there that have a similar situation and would love to stay physically fit and healthy by doing videos like these. If I could empower amputees to be active in a way that works for *them*, that would bring me so much fulfillment.

I realize that I may seem like a workout fanatic, but I'm not. I only workout 3-4 times a week and have my cheat days where I eat junk food and dessert, but for the most part, I am very health conscious. A part of that stems from knowing even the slightest weight gain or loss impacts the overall fit of my prosthesis. I have to be regimented. It's a great excuse and motivator to stay my current weight. I also know that the heavier I am, the more stress it puts on my knee. Weight management and exercise are ways that I combat the arthritis that is already beginning to infiltrate.

I've also noticed that I'm not able to put as much pressure on the bulbous end of my stump anymore. Before, I could run on it for short spurts and could walk around on it endlessly without it hurting. I would be out of breath from the physical exertion well before the pain ever arrived. However, that's not the case now. On bad days, I can only walk a couple of steps before the pain is intolerable. On good days, I might be able to withstand a minute or two.

My husband and I just redid our house that we bought in April of 2017. We ripped up all the carpet and put down vinyl flooring throughout our entire main floor. At night, when I'm relaxing and remove my prosthesis, I have a hard time walking. I'm not exactly sure what has changed. Maybe atrophy is to blame again, but the portion that once was my heel is not providing me with the same cushion as before. Walking on carpet isn't a problem yet, but hard surfaces are definitely a different story. Now, when Bob and I are sitting on the couch in the living room after the kids have gone to bed and the dog needs to be let out, I ask him to do it. If I get hungry and want a snack, I have two options: go through the hassle of putting my leg back on or once again ask Bob to get it for me.

Seeing that I am a working mom with two young children, this might actually be more of a gift than a curse; it allows me to be lazy for once in my life. I'm sure it's not Bob's favorite thing to do, but he does it without complaint...most times.

Recently, on a trip to Great Wolf Lodge, the problem became even more apparent. Great Wolf Lodge has an amazing indoor water park. Bob and I thought it would be a great family winter activity, so we booked a night's stay at their lodge which included passes to the park.

Once there, we got our purple wristbands on that allowed us entrance into the water park, and we put our bathing suits on. I put the girls' life jackets on while Bob stood in line to get some towels. When we were finally ready, we spotted a couple of open chairs to set down our belongings and my prosthesis so that we could keep everything off the ground in hopes of it staying dry.

Eliza was so excited to play in the little fountains that they had in the wave pool, so we decided to go to that section first. I sat down next to Eliza in the shallow, zero entry area while Bob took Gabriella into the deeper water so that she could have fun being tossed around by the waves. Since Eliza seemed so content where she was, I asked Bob to take Gabriella down one of the water slides. I knew there was no way that I could climb all the stairs leading up to the slides without my leg on. If I wore my prosthesis up there, then I would have to take it off at the top, go down the slide, and then go all the way back up and down the stairs to retrieve it. The stairs are a nightmare anyways because a huge line forms on them, so getting through the massive amount of people would be quite the task. Therefore, going down the slides was a Bob thing.

However, right when the two of them left, Eliza started getting more adventurous. She wasn't even two yet and had no clue how to swim, so I was on edge to say the least. Flashbacks of me being alone with Gabriella that day at the pool a few years ago came to mind.

Eliza ventured further away from me to the point where I was uncomfortable, which forced me to hobble over to her and sit back down in a new spot. She probably did that same thing ten different times. It was tiring, but the hard surface of the pool wasn't helping things either; every single step was painful. At one point, Eliza was faster than I thought and got to a relatively deep area. I frantically hurried to get up and run after her. My heart was pounding for fear that I wasn't going to get there in time. I got close enough to grab onto the strap that was attached to the back of the infant life jacket that she was wearing.

To say she was upset at being restrained is an understatement. She is such an independent child, so she wanted nothing to do with me holding her back from doing what she wanted to do. Right then and there, she decided to throw a full-blown fit. She laid on her stomach with her face down in the water and started flailing her arms and legs. I quickly turned her over and scooped her up in my arms, reprimanding her the entire way back to the shallow area.

I knew it wasn't safe to stay in the water without Bob's help (especially with me so physically exhausted), so after I got Eliza calmed down, the two of us held hands as we walked back to our chairs to take a break. I wrapped her in a towel and had her sitting on my lap while my mind started to shift to all of the "what if's." One of my flaws is overestimating my abilities. Because I am so stubborn and determined, sometimes I don't realize when I'm in over my head. In that situation, I should have been more cautious. There is a fine line, though, between holding myself back and overestimating, and sometimes it's hard to know what direction to go. I don't want to say "I can't" to things involving my leg, but this scenario showed me that when others' safety is concerned, I should.

189

After Bob and Gabriella got back from the slides, I told Bob what had happened.

"Why don't you sit here and take a break then? I will take them to the splash pad area," he suggested.

I reluctantly agreed. I can't even go in that area because of all the water that sprays. As I sat there by myself, I started feeling a little sorry for myself. All I wanted was to be with my family and enjoy our time together. When looking around at all the other people, I saw how capable they were. They walked around with ease, not having to worry about being able to chase their children or figure out how they were going to get around. Tears started coming to my eyes out of sheer frustration. I was angry that my leg was holding me back, jealous of the "normal people," and sad that I couldn't engage with my kids the same way other parents were. These feelings don't happen often, and even when it did happen, I was able to suppress them quickly, but not quick enough...

I had been caught. Bob was returning with the girls and could see all of the emotions that I was desperately trying to hide.

"You ok?" he asked.

"I guess," I replied.

"You're doing great, Kendra."

"But that's the thing—I'm not. Compared to other amputees, yeah, but to all these other people, no. I just want to play with my kids."

"I know, but look around. Half of the parents are on their cell phone and not interacting with their children at all. They're clear across the park, nowhere near them. Some of the other ones are downing beers and just talking to their friends. I promise you that you're doing better than them."

It was the reassurance that I needed. Bob doesn't sugar coat things; he calls them like he seems them. So, when he says something like that, I trust that he's being honest rather than just telling me what I want to hear.

Trying to keep the mood light, I asked Gabriella, "Are you having fun?"

"Oh yeah! Can we do the lazy river next?"

I looked at Bob, unsure.

"What do you think? You up for it?"

"Yeah, I think so. Should I put my leg on to go over there?" The lazy river was clear on the other side of the water park.

"I don't know where you would put it once we got over there. There aren't any chairs to put it on. I'll help you," he said as he held out his arm.

"I'll just hop," I said. But, after hopping about halfway, I needed to stop and rest. When I had caught my breath, I started walking on my stump to give my left leg a break. But, because I already put so much pressure on it earlier in the wave pool, I wasn't even able to take a few steps without being overcome with pain. Each time I put my full weight on the bulbous end of my stump, it felt like I was walking on needles. The pain was so bad that my leg completely gave out, and I couldn't help but cry out. I was able to catch myself by stepping up onto my left leg again, which kept me from falling down.

After hearing me cry out in pain, Gabriella said, "You can do it, Momma. Here, hold my hand." It was adorable to hear her encouragement. I know she didn't understand everything that I was going through and how hard it was for me, but the fact that she tried to ease the burden in her own five-year-old way was endearing.

I grabbed onto anything that I could to help me get from point A to point B. There were ropes that lined most of the areas, so I clutched onto them with my right arm in order to brace myself, helping take some of the pressure off my good leg.

When I finally got over to the lazy river, I got onto a raft and Bob put Eliza on my lap. It was nice to relax as we floated along with the current (except for the occasional bucket of water that was dumped on my head).

After the lazy river, Gabriella spotted an obstacle course that she wanted to try. I told Bob that I could sit on a half wall right by it and keep watch easily, so he took Eliza to the toddler area that had smaller slides. Right when it was her turn, Gabriella turns to me and says, "I have to go to the bathroom."

"Are you serious? Can you wait?" I asked.

"No. I have to go right now."

I looked around to find out where they were. Of course, they were on the opposite side of the park. I questioned letting her pee in the water but knew that would set the wrong precedent. "Well, come on then. They're right over there," I said as I pointed to the sign. "You go ahead. I'll follow behind, but it's gunna take me awhile, and I don't want you to have an accident." At that point, I couldn't bear to put any more pressure on my stump. It had taken all it could. The only option that I had was to hop... a really long distance. Thankfully, Bob and Eliza were right by the bathrooms, so we met up with them afterwards.

Gabriella is pretty self-sufficient in the water, especially with a life jacket on, so Bob and I decided to tag team Eliza going down the slide. Bob walked her up to the top of the slide while I waited in the water for her to come down. I snatched her up and guided her halfway to the steps until Bob could come and get her to repeat the process. After doing that about twenty times, I looked at Bob and said, "I'm sorry, but I just can't do it anymore. My left leg is killing me from working double time. We need to go."

Right as I said that, my left quadricep started to cramp. I made my way out of the pool and sat in a chair that was nearby. Meanwhile, Bob went and got my prosthesis so that I wouldn't have to walk all the way over to where our belongings were. As I was sitting there waiting for him to return, a woman was walking in my direction and seemed to lose her balance. She ran directly into me, accidentally scratching me with her fingernails. After she apologized profusely, I looked down and saw that something was wrong with her foot; it was turned inward, and she walked with a severe limp. I subtly continued to watch her as she entered the pool. When she was about knee deep, she tripped again and did a belly smack into the water. Nothing appeared to be hurt other than her pride, but as the events unraveled around me, I started feeling guilty for how I reacted earlier. I was naive and self-indulgent to think that I was the only one there with problems or physical limitations. Not that I enjoyed seeing her struggle, but it was nice to know that I wasn't alone in my challenges. Maybe it was some divine

192

intervention or a crazy coincidence, but either way, I'm glad it was me that she bumped into that day.

Unfortunately, things didn't get any easier after leaving the water park. As I walked to our room at the lodge, I could tell I was in for a rough couple of days. I already hurt and didn't even want to think about how stiff I was going to be in the morning. After the girls went to bed, I took some Ibuprofen and Bob gave me an hour-long massage to try to ease the pain. At that point, my whole body hurt. My back and left leg were the worst by far, but I could feel it everywhere. I felt like I had aged decades in the matter of one day.

It took me three days to recover from that trip. I'm sure it would have been hard on me either way, but I think it would have been a little easier if I could have walked on my stump more. Hopping from place to place was just too much for me. Needless to say, I don't think there will be too many more trips to water parks in the near future. Maybe when the kids get a little older and don't need me to be quite as vigilant, we'll have a redo.

The severity of the water park situation got me a little nervous about what my future holds. Will I eventually be at the point where I won't be weight bearing at all? Will I start to feel that same pain when I walk *with* my prosthesis? If so, I know that means I will be confined to a wheelchair or will have to use crutches. I start to wonder: When will I start needing assistance when getting into the shower? Will I have to stop driving or alter my car so that I can operate it? Will I be able to play sports with my kids or walk the dog?

I try to take things one day at a time, but on the occasion that I allow my mind to wander to those hypothetical scenarios, I get down. No matter what, our bodies degenerate as we age. I just fear that that might happen a little quicker for me than it does everyone else. But, there's only so much I can do to control those things. For now, I'm grateful for all the things that I *can* do.

Chapter 17

Hopes for the Future

I tend to dream big, and most of the time I'm stubborn enough to make those dreams into a reality. Of course, some of those dreams are selfish. I hope for things in the prosthetic world to get better and progress so that it can benefit *me*.

With technology progressing so quickly these days, it makes me excited for the impending changes. Things have changed a lot in the last thirty years, but with such technological momentum, I'm left to wonder what my prosthesis will look like in ten years. Will my skin look even more realistic? Will it allow for more versatility? Will it somehow be able to give me a smoother, more natural gate?

I recently got a post card in the mail from Optimus Prosthetics that highlighted an amputee's experience with a new, innovative practice. The card boasts that, "The Symphonie Aqua System allows practitioners to capture an accurate impression of the limb in weight-bearing, simulating a real-life experience for the patient." It also says that it would help them to "know about sensitive and problem areas before the socket is created to facilitate greater comfort and patient satisfaction." What a novel concept. I have only ever been casted while sitting down. So much changes when I put my full weight on my stump, so I imagine that using the Symphonie Aqua System might yield better results.

Advancements like this give me hope that my dream of having a water leg could one day come true. Maybe in the near future I could go down the biggest slide at the water park with my kids. I could take a walk on the beach without having to run up toward the shore to avoid a wave. I could even go snorkeling while wearing *two* flippers.

Insurance companies don't deem water legs as a *need*, so they don't typically fund them. However, what if that changed? Making water legs more accessible to the nearly two million people suffering from limb loss across America would be a game changer. When I talked to Eric Miller at The Shriners Medical Center, he said that water legs are highly requested. It makes perfect sense. What kid doesn't want to play in the water with his/her friends when it's 90 degrees outside? But, Eric went on to say that water legs are seen as a novelty, so they are often denied. He said that only kids who have a bigger need for them get approved. For example, Eric recently worked with a high school competitive swimmer. Because she was using the water leg for more than just leisure, he was able to grant her request.

I know the main concern is to provide a comfortable, functional prosthesis. But with all the advanced technology out there now, it's disappointing that water legs and other devices that are seen as "extras" couldn't be more accessible to the general populace.

- - -

However, it's not all about maximum comfort, nifty new gadgets, and water legs that would benefit *me*. I have always hoped to inspire others and make it easier for other amputees by sharing my story and little tricks that I've learned along the way (especially to new amputees who might need a bit more encouragement).

There is definitely a camaraderie that exists between amputees. When I see other amputees out in public, I feel called to go up and talk to them. It's important to have that support and commonality so we don't start to feel isolated. A few months ago, I was shopping at Walmart, and a man and his young daughter were in the same aisle as me as I shopped for shoes for my own daughters. I saw the man look down at my leg and then up at me. I could sense his hesitation as he decided whether or not he wanted to engage in conversation. Finally, he spoke: "Hi. I notice you have a prosthetic. Where do you have yours made?"

At first, I was kind of confused. Neither he nor his daughter seemed to have any trouble with their arms or legs. "I get mine at Optimus Prosthetics. It's located in Norwood."

"That's good to know. My son is scheduled to have his leg amputated very soon. He'll eventually need a prosthesis when everything is healed."

"Oh, I'm so sorry to hear that," I said. "If you don't mind me asking, why does he have to get it amputated?"

"He has cancer."

"Oh my gosh. That must be so hard."

"Well, it is what it is. What else can we do? There's no sense dwelling on it. We're just going to make the best of it," he said.

I admired his mindset, but my heart broke for him. Not wanting to pity them, I kept the conversation more upbeat. "Well, the good news is that it's happening when he's young. He will probably be able to do all sorts of things. Kids are resilient. I can run, swim, and do anything I put my mind to. I would recommend you looking into The Shriner's Medical Center in Lexington though. They will help you with the cost, and they did a great job with my prostheses when I was a kid."

I'm not sure what ever came of that family's situation. Maybe the dad wanted reassurance or to simply just talk to another amputee. Either way, I hope he could see the possibilities and opportunities for his son by seeing how well I have adjusted.

-   -   -

Similarly, last year Bob and I went to a Cincinnati Red's baseball game. About halfway through the game, Bob tapped me on the shoulder and leaned in to whisper, "Do you see that man about five rows in front of us? He's an amputee."

I looked down and saw a man wearing camo shorts, a black t-shirt, and a Red's hat. Both of his arms were covered in tattoos. I didn't think much more about it until he left his seat and started climbing the stairs during the seventh inning stretch. Despite his muscular build, he was really struggling to make his way up. As typical, Bob flagged him down and struck up a conversation.

"Hey, my wife is an amputee," he said, pointing at me. "Do you mind me asking how you lost your leg?"

"Oh, sure," he said as he sat down on the stair beside Bob. "I lost it almost a year ago when I was serving in Iraq. An IED went off."

"Oh man, I'm sorry to hear that. How are things going for you now?"

"Well, I've been through four sockets in less than a year. Every time the swelling goes down and my leg changes, I have to get a new one. It's still very painful, and I'm not really used to it yet."

"Man, that's gotta be tough," Bob said sympathetically.

"Yeah, but I'm alive." He shrugged his shoulders and let out a little sigh.

They talked for a while longer about the military. Bob has quite a few family members that have served or are currently serving, so they had a lot of stories to share. At the end of the conversation, Bob said, "You still heading up there?" He pointed towards the snack vendors.

"Yeah," he said.

"Well, I'll go with ya. I'll buy you a beer."

After listening in on their conversation, I had a lot of conflicting emotions. I was empathetic, but I also felt guilty. I could do so many things that he couldn't yet do. But, on top of that, there was also a disconnect. I should have been able to interject in the conversation and say, "Yeah, I know what you're feeling." But, I couldn't really relate to any part of his story other than adjusting to a new prosthesis. Losing a limb later in life is not something that I've experienced, nor do I know about the emotional toll going to war had on him (or anyone else for that matter). But again, just like the family in Walmart, I hope that I could provide some hope or encouragement to the veteran that day. Maybe by seeing how well I could get around, it gave him the inspiration that he needed to keep pushing through and the strength to endure the hardships that he encountered throughout his journey of healing.

Additionally, in listing my desires to help and inspire others, I would be remiss if I didn't include writing this book. In fact, it's the *sole* reason that I'm writing it. A few months before my mom died, she told me that she couldn't wait for God to tell her whose lives she had impacted over the years. She said that we never know the breadth of our influence. I may never know if someone was inspired, gained courage or hope, became stronger, or started to change their mentality because of my book. But, if one person was changed for the better because of it, then this whole process was worth it.

- - -

Besides my selfish desire to reap the benefits of advancing technology and aiming to inspire others, it is my hope that society continues to become more accepting and further embrace people who are considered "different." We have certainly come a long way. In recent years, the media (and people in general) have made great strides to be more sensitive.

For example, I was shopping at Walmart on a different occasion in search of a toy for my daughter. As I perused the aisles, something caught my eye. I stopped dead in my tracks when I saw a large doll that wore a prosthesis. Although I was pleased by just seeing an amputee represented in a doll, there was more to it than that. The company who made the doll really put thought into how they would portray her. She was not only an amputee, but a gymnast. The icing on the cake was the gold medal that adorned her neck. The doll was depicted as strong, capable, and talented. What a great message to send to the general public; people with physical limitations can still accomplish so much!

You should have seen Gabriella's face when I gave her the doll. The first words out of her mouth were, "Momma, it looks exactly like you!" What a difference having a doll like that could have made for me when I was a child.

"Do you know what you're going to name her," I asked.

There was no hesitation. "Kendra," she said.

"You're going to name her after me? That's awesome," I told her, beaming with pride.

Later that night, we went to Bob's school's football game. Gabriella took the doll to the game and wouldn't let it out of her sight. One of Bob's coworkers named Andrea came up to us.

After we made small talk for a while, Andrea noticed what Gabriella was holding. "I like your doll," she said.

"Thanks. I named it Kendra because it has a prosthesis like my mom. Look, her leg even comes off!" she said as she pulled off the doll's blue, plastic prosthesis.

"Oh my gosh. That's so neat! I didn't even notice her leg." There was a brief pause in the conversation. Andrea's eyes welled up with tears. "Girl, you made me cry," she said, dabbing her eyes.

Gabriella was too young to understand what warranted Andrea's tears. That instance illuminated Gabriella's innocence. She was blind to the doll's imperfections, which I knew could be extended to me. She saw me as beautiful and whole. There's no better type of love that that—unconditional, unadulterated, pure.

I was so enamored with the doll that I went home that night and posted a picture of it on Facebook. One of my friends commented on it and asked if I had heard about the new Barbie line that Mattel was unveiling. The caption of the picture she sent me boasted, "The new 2019 Barbie Fashionistas line from Mattel will feature a doll in a wheelchair and another with a prosthetic leg."

With this type of progress, people with physical limitations can hopefully start to have a better self-image. No longer are we forced to compare ourselves to the perfect body type. People like us exist not only in reality but also on the shelves. Physically challenged children can play with dolls that look like them. But not only that, kids with no physical impairments think it's cool too! What child wouldn't enjoy taking off his doll's leg? It's interactive, new, and different. It's steps like this that leave me hopeful for a more accepting and loving future.

- - -

Eric Miller told me in our interview, "I can build the best prosthesis, but if the patient has a bad attitude, they won't walk well. It's a mindset." I can't help but agree with him. People with physical limitations are faced with a daily choice: fight or give up. When comparing the two life paths, the first option will likely yield a more gratifying life. Having come to that conclusion, I try every day to have a fighter's mentality.

However, society can make all these positive strides, but in the end, it won't matter if the individual doesn't have the mental fortitude needed to thrive. Who would have thought that I would be able to do more with less? Probably not many. But, ironically, removing a part of me made me more whole.

It took me years to embrace who I am and become mentally strong enough to deal with the emotional side of being an amputee. Even still, there are days where I feel sorry for myself or my confidence wavers. But, I know I have grown because when people refer to me as disabled or handicapped, I no longer correct them. In fact, I take it as a compliment—a badge that I proudly display. I am more than my disability, but I am still an amputee. It is just as much a part of me as any other trait I possess, and I wouldn't have it any other way.

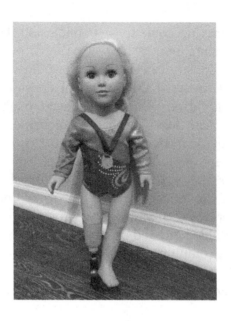

My daughter, Gabriella, named this doll after me because of its artificial leg and blonde hair.

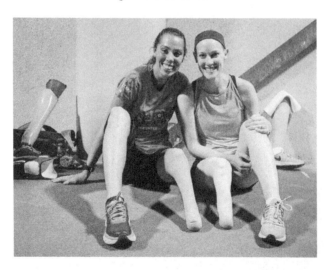

Grace Norman, Olympic Gold Medalist in the Triathlon, and I at a running clinic that she put on with the help of Optimus Prosthetics (photo credit: Rob McCulley).

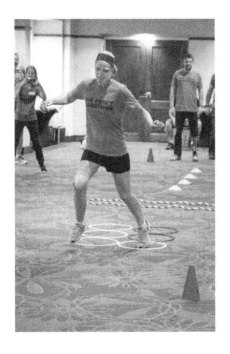

All the amputees that attended the running clinic ended the day with a friendly obstacle course competition. We took turns racing Grace Norman, but inevitably she beat us all.

Epilogue

There are two qualities that I have noticed in myself lately that I also see becoming a problem in others. The first one is the tendency to avoid negative or difficult situations at all costs. If you're anything like me, when things get hard, you try to find a way to skirt around it. I often try to soften the blow to make it easier, so I don't have to feel the negative emotions. It's a natural defense mechanism that many of us innately have. But, what if we're meant to *feel* the pain? To embrace it even? We need the grit and tenacity that those hardships help us develop, but, even though I'm aware of it, I go to great lengths to protect myself and remain comfortable.

However, in remaining comfortable, we don't grow. Don't get me wrong, it's really difficult to remember that in the moment. But, I never want to forget that life is hard sometimes. No matter how sorry I feel for myself or how much I want to throw in the towel on my bad days, I always want to remain grateful for what becoming an amputee has taught me, and more importantly, what it's made me. God has used my deformity to make me a stronger, more compassionate person. Plus, if I hadn't experienced the hardships, I wouldn't know how good I have it or be appreciative when things are going well.

I challenge you to try to do the same. The next time you run into an obstacle or an unpleasant situation, try not to give in to your natural tendency to avoid it and run the other way. Instead, focus on what it can teach you or what it's doing to develop your character. You might have the same outcome that I've had—personal growth. If nothing else, you'll be a happier person with a better outlook on life.

The second quality that I've noticed about myself is not wanting to offend anyone. We live in the era of political correctness, and I'm no different; I'm a people pleaser by nature. Although it has helped me in a lot of facets of my life, it has made me shy away from certain situations. When I see someone in a wheelchair or someone with a physical limitation, I sometimes look away. I don't want that person to think that I'm staring. Maybe it's because I'm uncomfortable with him/her being different than me, but often it's because I don't want to be offensive.

About a month ago, my family and I went to Bob's hometown to visit. We all decided to go to his parents' church on Saturday night. At the end of mass, one of Bob's friends from high school came up to us to say hi. I was talking to Bob's parents when I felt a tap on my shoulder.

"Hey Kendra," Bob said, "I want you to meet Dwight. I went to high school with him."

When I turned around, I saw a man in a wheelchair. Not knowing what his limitations were, the first thing that came to my mind was *I know it's polite to shake hands, but what if he doesn't have the ability to do so?* Because I felt uncomfortable and I didn't want to offend him or make *him* uncomfortable, I didn't shake his hand. Instead, I did some stupid little wave and said hello.

Of all people, I should have known better. I've dealt with the same thing my whole life. People stare at me, but they rarely ask what happened. I know they don't want to offend me or bring up a touchy subject, but what many people don't realize is that I would love to talk about my leg and inform other people about it. Staring is normal. Who wouldn't stare at something that is different or intriguing? People aren't staring to be mean. They're just curious. Bob is always getting upset when people stare at me, but I welcome it. People *should* take a few seconds to observe and learn about each other. However, I challenge that we should follow up those stares with a conversation full of questions.

I know I have a lot of room to grow in dealing with people who are different than me. Interacting with Dwight made that even more apparent. I didn't even give him an appropriate greeting. How belittling and rude! It's ironic that I was striving so hard to not offend him, but in the end, I offended him by not shaking his hand.

If you can learn anything from my mistake, treat other people like *people*. Don't be the type to put fake hands in pools and taunt people by calling them "pirate" or "one-legged whore" just because looking at them makes you a little uncomfortable. Worry less about offending them and more about being a friend and being kind. And, when things feel awkward or uncomfortable, don't let that be your excuse for avoiding them. I can guarantee you that they're probably feeling ten times more self-conscious than you. Knowing that it was harder for me to feel comfortable in my skin than it was for a lot of other people, take the first step and reach out to people who are different than you. Who knows, maybe initiating a conversation will make their day and break the ice enough to ensure both parties are comfortable.

Visit my website to view more pictures, read some of my poetry, and catch up on updates: https://kendraherber.wixsite.com/mysite

Acknowledgements

Bob- Thank you for: loving me *because* I'm different, for your encouragement and patience through the writing process, for letting me dream and believing in me, for acting as another editor by scrutinizing every. single. sentence. of this book, and for helping raise our daughters to believe that there is beauty in all types of people. I love you!

Melanie Monahan- Thank you for designing a beautiful cover and letting me have control over everything while still letting you work your magic. Your talent and artistic vision still amaze me.

Mackenzie Ludwig- Thank you for editing my entire novel at NO COST. Please know that I will never forget your selflessness and generosity. This book wouldn't be half as good without your feedback.

Robert McCulley- You are another one that provided your services for free! You take beautiful pictures, but you have an even bigger heart.

Rachel McChesney and Jackie Oldiges- Thank you for being my springboard and for listening to me drone on and on about the book. I appreciate you acting like you cared even when I talked way too much about it. Jackie, your feedback and corrections were much appreciated and brought more emotion and life to my book. I still think that with your intelligence and writing ability, *you* should have written this book instead... if only you were an amputee.

Dad and Aunt Joyce- Thanks for supplying me with a part of my story that I never even knew existed. That was the best part of writing this book- it made me ask questions about my early years that I never would have thought to ask. I now feel like my story is complete.

Mom- Thanks for fostering my love of writing at an early age. Even when my writing was terrible, you made me think it was the best thing ever written. The words that you wrote to me in a letter just before you died meant more to me than you will ever know and inspired me to tackle a feat as big as writing my own memoir: "Kendra, I have seen how your creative writing has been an outlet for you to express some of your deepest emotions. It would be fantastic if one day you got published, but I don't think that would change the impact your poems have on you and those who do read them. Thank you for sharing some of them with me." Thanks for reminding me that being published doesn't matter, but my words do.

Optimus Prosthetics and The Shriner's Medical Center- Thank you for always supplying me with the best care. You have exceeded my expectations in so many ways. Thanks for putting up with how high maintenance I am and always remaining patient. I can't tell you how much I appreciate you trying new things, being resourceful, and doing so much research to provide me with such wonderful products. Thanks for making your job feel like more of a passion.